# Neurologic Localization and Diagnosis

# Neurologic Localization and Diagnosis

**Karl E. Misulis, M.D., Ph.D.**
*Neurologist, Semmes–Murphey Clinic, Jackson, Tennessee;
Associate Clinical Professor of Neurology, Vanderbilt
University School of Medicine, Nashville, Tennessee*

**Butterworth–Heinemann**

Boston   Oxford   Johannesburg   Melbourne   New Delhi   Singapore

**Library of Congress Cataloging-in-Publication Data**
Misulis, Karl E.
    Neurologic localization and diagnosis / Karl E. Misulis.
        p.   cm.
    Includes index.
    ISBN: 0-7506-9636-2 (alk. paper)
        1.  Nervous systems—Diseases—Diagnosis—Handbooks, manuals, etc.
    2.  Brain—Localization of functions—Handbooks, manuals, etc.   3.  Physical
    diagnosis—Handbooks, manuals, etc.   4.  Medical history taking—Handbooks,
    manuals, etc.   I.  Title.
    (DNLM:   1.  Nervous Systems Diseases—diagnosis—handbooks.
    WL 39 M678n   1996]
    RC348.M53   1996
    616.8′0475—dc20
    DNLM/DLC
    for Library of Congress                                              95-50501
                                                                              CIP


**British Library Cataloguing-in-Publication Data**
A catalogue record for this book is available from the British Library.


The publisher offers discounts on bulk orders of this book.
For information, please write:
Manager of Special Sales
Butterworth–Heinemann
313 Washington Street
Newton, MA 02158-1626

10 9 8 7 6 5 4 3 2 1

Printed in the United States of America

# Contents

*Preface*                                               ix
*Abbreviations*                                         xi


**1. Cerebral Cortex and White Matter**                **1**
Anatomy                                                  1
   Functional Localization                1
   Pathological Localization              7
Motor and Sensory Dysfunction                           33
   Weakness                               33
   Sensory Loss                           34
   Apraxia                                35
   Akinesia                               38
Aphasia                                                 39
Dementia                                                42
Visual Field Abnormalities                              46
Visuospatial Dysfunction                                49

**2. Basal Ganglia and Thalamus**                      **51**
Basal Ganglia                                           51
   Anatomy                                51
   Lesions                                54
Thalamus                                                65
   Anatomy                                65
   Lesions                                67

### 3. Cranial Nerves, Brain Stem, and Cerebellum       71

Cranial Nerves                                              71
   Olfactory Nerve                           71
   Optic Nerve                               74
   Ocular Motor System                       75
   Trigeminal Nerve                          94
   Facial Nerve                              95
   Vestibulocochlear Nerve                   99
   Glossopharyngeal Nerve                    102
   Vagus                                     103
   Accessory Nerve                           105
   Hypoglossal Nerve                         106
Brain Stem                                                 107
   Overview                                  107
   Midbrain                                  112
   Pons                                      115
   Medulla                                   118
Cerebellum                                                 120
   Anatomy                                   120
   Lesions                                   121
Cranial Nerve, Brain Stem, and Cerebellar
  Syndromes                                       127
   Arnold–Chiari Malformation                127
   Dandy–Walker Syndrome                     128
   Foster–Kennedy Syndrome                   128
   Cavernous Sinus Syndrome                  129
   Tolosa–Hunt Syndrome                      129
   Superior Orbital Fissure Syndrome         129
   Cerebellopontine Angle Syndrome           129
   Gradenigo's Syndrome                      130
   Basilar Thrombosis                        130
   Olivopontocerebellar Atrophy and Multiple
    System Atrophy                       131
   Shy–Drager Syndrome                       131
   Top-of-the-Basilar Syndrome               132

**4. Spinal Cord**      **133**

Anatomy      133
  Segmental Anatomy      133
  Tracts      133
  Vascular Anatomy of the Spinal Cord      138
Lesions      138
  Guide to Localization      138
  Tumors Affecting the Spinal Cord      141
  Brown–Séquard Syndrome      142
  Tabes Dorsalis and Syphilitic Myelitis      143
  Transverse Myelitis      143
  Multiple Sclerosis      144
  Syringomyelia      144
  Anterior Horn Cell Disease      145
  Vascular Disease      147
  Lesions at Specific Spinal Levels      149

**5. Peripheral Nerve and Muscle**      **155**

Anatomy      155
Examination      157
Differential Diagnosis of Neuromuscular Disorders      159
  Nerve Conduction Velocity and Electromyography
    Interpretation      159
  Muscle and Nerve Biopsy      161
  Laboratory Tests      162
Neuropathies      163
  Differential Diagnosis      163
  Polyneuropathies      167
  Mononeuropathies      172
  Mononeuropathy Multiplex      181
  Motoneuron Disease      181
Myopathies      182
  Dystrophies      182
  Inflammatory Myopathies      182
  Metabolic Myopathies      184

Periodic Paralysis  184
Endocrine Myopathies  187
Neuromuscular Transmission Defects  188
Myasthenia Gravis  189
Botulism  189
Myasthenic (Eaton–Lambert) Syndrome  189

*Appendix*  *191*

*Index*  *201*

# Preface

The key to diagnosis of most neurologic disorders is anatomic localization. With some neurologic conditions, the diagnosis is occasionally obvious, but often the symptoms and signs do not fit a specific
syndrome. The clinician might arrive at the diagnosis by performing
all known functional and structural laboratory tests, but this approach would be expensive and unfair to the patient—and might
not even reveal the diagnosis.

This small book is a guide to the diagnosis of neurologic disorders, with an emphasis on localization through history and examination. Where appropriate, confirmatory laboratory tests are
discussed. For optimal use of this book, read it from cover to cover,
concentrating on the text and ignoring the details found in the figures and tables. Then stick it in your pocket, black bag, or car trunk
as a ready reference.

If this book aids in the efficient diagnosis of neurologic disorders, then my purpose has been accomplished.

KARL E. MISULIS

# Abbreviations

| | |
|---|---|
| ACA | anterior cerebral artery |
| ACh | acetylcholine |
| AChR | acetylcholine receptor |
| AD | Alzheimer's disease |
| ADM | abductor digiti minimi |
| AICA | anterior inferior cerebellar artery |
| ALS | amyotrophic lateral sclerosis |
| ANA | antinuclear antibody |
| APB | abductor pollicus brevis |
| CIDP | chronic inflammatory demyelinating polyradiculoneuropathy |
| CK | creatine kinase |
| CMAP | compound motor action potential |
| CMT | Charcot–Marie–Tooth disease |
| CN | cranial nerve |
| CNS | central nervous system |
| CP | cerebral palsy |
| CPT | carnitine palmityltransferase |
| CSF | cerebrospinal fluid |
| CT | computerized tomography |
| DTR | deep tendon reflex |
| EAC | external auditory canal |
| ECS | electrocerebral silence |
| EEG | electroencephalography |
| EMG | electromyography |
| EP | evoked potential |
| ESR | erythrocyte sedimentation rate |
| ET | essential tremor |
| FDP | flexor digitorum profundus |
| GBS | Guillain–Barré syndrome |
| GI | gastrointestinal |
| HD | Huntington's disease |
| HIV | human immunodeficiency virus |

| | |
|---|---|
| HMSN | hereditary motor–sensory neuropathy |
| HSV | herpes simplex virus |
| IAC | internal auditory canal |
| ICP | intracranial pressure |
| IgG | immunoglobulin G |
| INO | internuclear ophthalmoplegia |
| LDH | lactate dehydrogenase |
| MCA | middle cerebral artery |
| MCP | metacarpal–phylangeal |
| MD | muscular dystrophy |
| MG | myasthenic gravis |
| MID | multi-infarct dementia |
| MLF | medial longitudinal fasciculus |
| MRI | magnetic resonance imaging |
| MS | multiple sclerosis |
| NADH–CoQ | nicotinamide adenine dinucleotide–coenzyme Q |
| NCV | nerve conduction velocity |
| OKN | optokinetic nystagmus |
| OPCA | olivopontocerebellar atrophy |
| PCA | posterior cerebral artery |
| PD | Parkinson's disease |
| PFK | phosphofructokinase |
| PICA | posterior inferior cerebellar artery |
| PIP | proximal interphylangeal |
| PMA | progressive muscular atrophy |
| PPRF | paramedian pontine reticular formation |
| RA | rheumatoid arthritis |
| SLE | systemic lupus erythematosus |
| SMA | spinal muscular atrophy |
| SNAP | sensory nerve action potential |
| TD | tardive dyskinesia |
| VA | ventral anterior |
| VL | ventrolateral |
| VP | ventroposterior |
| VPL | ventroposterolateral |
| VPM | ventroposteromedial |
| WBC | white blood cell |

# Cerebral Cortex and White Matter

## ANATOMY

Cerebral localization cannot be depicted simply by a labeled diagram of the brain. A specific location is frequently involved in multiple functions, and execution of one task requires multiple neural locations. As students of the body, we want to understand functional localization, that is, location of the neurons that participate in particular tasks. As physicians, however, we find pathological localization more clinically useful, since patients present with lesions that fall into pathophysiological patterns—for instance, left occipital lobe producing hemianopia or upper motoneuron degeneration producing spasticity.

### Functional Localization

#### *Language*

Language consists of receptive and expressive functions in conjunction with cognitive associations. Reception can be hearing or reading; expression can be speech or writing.

#### *Reception*

The first step to reception is function of the sensory organs, whether ears or eyes. For hearing, air waves are transduced into electrical signals by the elements of the middle ear and the cochlea. The acoustic nerve conducts the signal to the brain stem where it ascends bilaterally to the primary auditory cortex on the superior temporal gyrus (Heschl's gyrus). The auditory input is then translated into language content in Wernicke's area on the posterior aspect of the superior temporal gyrus, on the left side.

Reading is accomplished by receiving input from the visual cortex and decoding the information into language content. This is performed in the region of the angular gyrus on the inferior parietal lobule (Figure 1.1).

*Expression*

The first step toward expression is selection of the mode of output, whether through speech, writing, or other motor signals such as gestures and signing. Where concepts are synthesized into speech is unknown, but this probably does not happen in Broca's area. Broca's area, in the inferior frontal convolution, translates expressed language into commands that are executed by the motor cortex and descending systems for the creation of speech. Expression in writ-

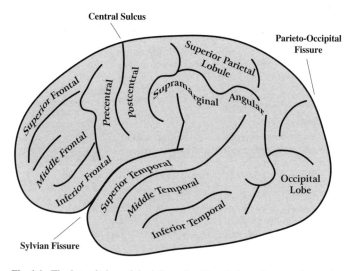

**Fig. 1.1** The lateral view of the left cerebral hemisphere shows major gyri and important landmarks.

ing is similar to expression in speech except that the motor commands are to the regions of the motor system concerning the arm and hand.

Repeating a received word requires input to the temporal lobe and relay of the information to the interior frontal region via the arcuate fasciculus, which passes beneath the angular and supramarginal gyri.

### *Vision*

The primary visual cortex is in the medial aspect of the occipital lobe on either side of the calcarine fissure (Figure 1.2). Cortex

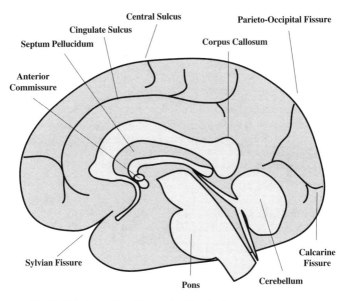

**Fig. 1.2**   Medial view of the right cerebral hemisphere.

above the fissure serves the lower-half field of vision, while cortex below the fissure serves the upper-half field of vision. Secondary visual areas are adjacent to the primary visual cortex and are involved in processing of visual information. Connections with other areas are responsible for even more complex associations; for example, connections between visual association areas with dominant hemisphere temporal lobes facilitate identification of visual symbols as words.

## Motor System

The precentral gyrus contains the pyramidal tract neurons that project to the brain stem and spinal cord to guide movement. Input to this area comes from many centers, including the frontal premotor region. Cortical and subcortical associative connections abound, as well. The premotor area probably contributes to initiation of movement. The precentral gyrus is topographically organized: lateral and inferior cortical areas represent the face and arm, and a parasagittal area represents the leg area on the precentral gyrus (Figure 1.3). Extensive frontal and parietal projections to the basal ganglia aid with control over movement.

## Somatosensory System

The somatosensory cortex is located on the postcentral gyrus, and it is topographically organized, as is the motor strip. Input comes from the thalamus; there are also associative connections with other cortical regions, including the motor cortex.

## Behavior and Affect

The pathways determining behavior and affect are so diffuse that they cannot be attributed to discrete anatomic locations. Although this section concerns normal anatomy rather than pathological correlations, most of the information on behavior comes from lesion studies.

Lesions of the left hemisphere are commonly associated with depression, whereas lesions of the right hemisphere can be associated with inappropriate cheerfulness. Rage can be seen with hypothalamic and temporal lobe lesions, and it is thought to result

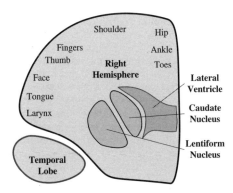

**Fig. 1.3** Coronal view of the left cerebral hemisphere at approximately the level of the central sulcus. The cortex is topographically organized in this region; anatomic regions served by the cortex are indicated.

from a defect in limbic system control over emotion. The abnormality associated with rage is not so much in the response but rather in the insignificance or absence of a trigger of the rage reaction.

Some patients with complex partial seizures have been described as having a "temporal lobe personality." This is a controversial concept in neurology. Many patients with complex partial seizures have a focus in the mesial temporal region, near the amygdala and hippocampus; the amygdala may be integrally involved in aggression. Components of the temporal lobe personality have been described as including hyposexuality, hyperreligiosity, hypergraphia (excessive writing), and obsessive behavior. Rare patients may manifest overly aggressive behavior. Violent attacks can be an ictal event, though the violence is not focused and premeditated in such cases; directed violence in patients with "temporal lobe personalities" is probably a manifestation of a personality disorder rather than an ictal event. It should be emphasized that the personality changes accompanying a temporal lobe disorder are uncommon and highly variable.

### Memory and Intellect

Most dementing illnesses affect the brain diffusely or are multifocal. Global deterioration in intellectual function usually means global neuronal dysfunction; however, the frontal and temporal lobes are more important than other regions for these functions.

The neuronal substrates of learning and memory remain under intense study, but we do know a little about the neuroanatomy of these functions. Dr. Frank Benson divides memory into three basic processes:

- Immediate recall
- Learning
- Retrieval

Immediate recall is accomplished by retrieval of sensory information stored in the neural matrix throughout the brain; both hemispheres are probably important for this process. The input to the brain is through the region responsible for the sensory modality: for instance, the primary auditory cortex is responsible for verbal information. The verbal information is then decoded by associative language regions into concepts that the individual can understand. If the subject is asked to repeat the information, the concepts are translated once again into language, then into the sequence of motor commands required to speak the answer. Immediate recall does not call on long-term memory; immediate recall has a short half-life and is especially susceptible to distraction.

Data to be remembered for longer than the time required for immediate recall are learned, which means that a longer-term storage mode for the information is formed. The molecular basis of this long-term storage is not known, but it is believed to involve the limbic system. The limbic system may be directly involved in establishing memory, or it may indirectly facilitate memory by assigning importance to pieces of information as they are processed in sensory association areas; that is, a piece of information perceived by the limbic system to have importance for the individual will be assigned a high priority for memory. Each hemisphere has all of the limbic components required, since surgical removal of one hemisphere has little effect on learning. This fact reinforces the notion that data are not stored directly in the temporal parts of the limbic system.

From experience with computers, we have a tendency to compartmentalize functions and storage sites. Fortunately, memory does not appear to be stored as scripts or pictures in focal areas of the brain. Long-term memory is more likely a complex interrelation of past experiences with current intellectual development. For example, the memory of a camping trip taken as a child could involve understanding the identity of a tent in the mind's encyclopedia, memories of family and friends who were (or could have been) on the trip, and perhaps recollection of a few scenes that were judged worthy of long-term storage. To these images is tied the emotional charge attached by a nostalgic mind reflecting on past times. Because of the complex interconnections of different parts of the brain required to establish this memory, a single focal area of infarction would be unlikely to erase total memory of this event. Unfortunately, however, this long-term storage is not always accurate, since the data are stored as concepts and impressions rather than as rote sensory experiences.

The mechanisms for retrieval are even less understood than those for learning. A triggering event must start the search process, whether an exogenous request for information or an introspective thought. The mind likely searches for components of the requested memory; when one part is found, the interconnections are then more easily established. This setup would explain how you might not recall a particular case at first, but then, on receiving sufficient information to trigger the memory, you would remember it in great detail.

**Pathological Localization**

Lesions of the cerebral hemispheres can be divided into three broad categories:

- Diffuse
- Multifocal
- Focal

### Diffuse Cerebral Lesions

Diffuse or global cerebral damage results in encephalopathy without focal neurologic findings. Important causes include anoxic and metabolic encephalopathy, some forms of encephalitis and toxins.

Diagnosis of diffuse disorders is aided by distinguishing whether the predominance of damage has occurred in cortical or subcortical tissue. Some pathological lesions affect the cerebral cortex and subcortical tissues approximately equally; others affect one more than the other. For example, Alzheimer's disease (AD), a neuronal degeneration, produces a prominent cortical dementia, whereas multiple sclerosis (MS), a white matter disorder, produces mainly subcortical damage. Table 1.1 lists distinguishing features of cortical and subcortical lesions and gives examples of each.

#### Anoxic Encephalopathy

Anoxic encephalopathy is one of the most common reasons for neurologic consultation in the hospital. Patients present with forms

**Table 1.1  Cortical versus Subcortical Lesions**

| Feature | Cortical | Subcortical |
|---|---|---|
| **Clinical features** | | |
| Dementia | Common | Common with advanced |
| Aphasia | Common | Uncommon |
| Ataxia | Uncommon | Common |
| **Personality change** | Common in early disease | Common in advanced disease |
| **Examples** | Alzheimer's and Picks disease, cortical infarctions | Multiple sclerosis, small-vessel infarctions |
| **Associated findings** | With multiple cortical infarctions, embolic etiology common | If cerebrovascular, cardiovascular disease common |

of encephalopathy ranging from mild cognitive impairment to profound coma. The role of evaluation is to identify the cause of encephalopathy and provide prognostic information.

Evaluation of the patient thought to have anoxic encephalopathy should answer the following questions:

- Is there a cause for the encephalopathy other than anoxic damage?
- Did a neurologic event such as seizure or stroke precipitate the anoxia?
- What is the level of dysfunction of the central nervous system (CNS)?
- How long has the encephalopathy been present?
- What changes have occurred since the precipitating event?

The search for causes of encephalopathy other than anoxia includes looking for additional factors, such as electrolyte imbalance, that can be corrected, allowing for improved neuronal function.

Determining the level of dysfunction is important for prognosis. First, the level of consciousness and the integrity of brain stem function are assessed. Profound impairment of consciousness and brain stem dysfunction point to a poor prognosis.

The examination should be comprehensive, and it should include specific attention to the following:

- Level of consciousness, including response to commands
- Pupil responses
- Eye movements
- Corneal responses

While assessing level of consciousness, subtle responses should be sought; for instance, eye movements may be the only sign of consciousness in locked-in syndrome. Within 24 hours, a poor prognosis is indicated by the following findings:

- No pupillary response
- No corneal response
- Absence of conjugate roving gaze

At one week following the anoxic event, a poor prognosis is indicated by the following findings:

- Absence of conjugate roving gaze
- Absence of spontaneous eye opening
- No response to commands

Evaluation of patients with anoxic encephalopathy must also include an accurate determination of the severity of anoxia and the duration of coma, if present. In general, longer anoxia and increased duration of coma indicate a poor prognosis for good neurologic recovery.

Electroencephalography (EEG) is often performed after anoxia to aid with prognosis. Electrocerebral silence (ECS) indicates a negligible chance of good neurologic recovery. Patterns associated with poor prognosis, although not as absolutely as ECS, include bilateral periodic discharges, repetitive sharp waves, spindle coma, alpha coma, and persistent triphasic waves. An EEG that is normal or shows mild slowing suggests that a good neurologic outcome is possible, but it in no way guarantees survival and recovery.

*Metabolic and Toxic Encephalopathy*
Encephalopathy is a very common reason for neurologic consultation in the hospital. The patient with encephalopathy often is hospitalized for any of numerous problems, including cancer, fever, elevated blood pressure, worsening renal function, bleeding due to coagulation disorders, or weakness. Before or during hospitalization, the patient develops confusion, sometimes associated with agitation or somnolence. No focal neurologic signs may be noted. The purpose of examination is to determine the reason for the encephalopathy. Unfortunately, clinical examination may not be of much help in establishing the etiology. While possible causes are numerous, the following should be considered:

TOXINS
- Drugs, prescribed and nonprescribed
- Ethanol intoxication
- Ethanol withdrawal
- Heavy metals

METABOLIC CAUSES
- Renal failure
- Hepatic failure
- Hyponatremia
- Hypernatremia
- Hypercalcemia
- Hypocalcemia
- Hypoglycemia
- Hyperglycemia
- Hypomagnesemia (usually with other electrolyte disorders)

ENDOCRINE CAUSES
- Hypothyroidism
- Hyperthyroidism
- Cushing's syndrome

NUTRITIONAL CAUSES
- Wernicke's encephalopathy
- Vitamin $B_{12}$ deficiency
- Nicotinic acid deficiency
- Possible folate deficiency

RESPIRATORY CAUSES
- Hypoxia
- Hypercarbia

Evaluation of patients with suspected encephalopathy begins with a thorough examination of the chart, including prescribed drugs and results of laboratory studies. Particular attention is paid to electrolyte derangements and abnormalities in renal and/or hepatic function. Thiamine is administered to virtually all patients, even in the absence of a documented history of ethanol abuse, for two reasons: (1) Ethanol abuse is often unreported; (2) Wernicke's encephalopathy can develop in the absence of ethanol abuse. Cancer patients and patients with nutritional deficiency develop symptoms of thiamine deficiency more often than is recognized. Important drugs associated with encephalopathy include the following:

- *Sedatives and hypnotics.* Benzodiazepines, especially those with active metabolites (such as diazepam), are commonly associated with encephalopathy.
- *Tricyclic antidepressants.* Amitriptyline, which is commonly prescribed for sedation at night, has a frequent hangover effect, especially in the elderly. All anticholinergic drugs should be avoided in the elderly and in patients with an organic brain syndrome.
- *Analgesics.* While almost any analgesic can be a problem, propoxyphene, meperidine, hydrocodone, codeine, and oxycodone are commonly associated with encephalopathy. Meperidine should not be used long-term because of buildup of active metabolites.
- *Miscellaneous*: H1 and H2 blockers and certain antipsychotic agents have been implicated in encephalopathy.

*Cerebral Palsy*
Cerebral palsy (CP) is a motor disorder due to brain damage during gestation or birth. Strictly used, CP indicates a nonprogressive disorder. Common causes are trauma and hypoxia, but the cause is not identified in many patients; erroneous assumption of negligent obstetric care often leads to inappropriate lawsuits. CP-related damage can be divided into the following categories:

- Neuronal necrosis
- Basal ganglia dysfunction
- Watershed infarcts
- Focal infarcts and trauma
- Periventricular hemorrhage

*Neuronal necrosis:*  Neuronal necrosis occurs with hypoxia or extensive trauma and is characterized by widespread neuronal degeneration. Patients present with spastic quadriplegia, mental retardation, and seizures.

*Basal ganglia dysfunction:*  Basal ganglia dysfunction is prominent in some patients with CP. Patients present with choreoathetosis and dystonia and may have relative preservation of intellectual function. Basal ganglia dysfunction is discussed further in Chapter 2.

*Watershed infarcts:* Watershed infarcts are usually caused by hypotension. Damage is most prominent in regions that do not have a rich vascular supply, often the border zones between major arterial distributions; the posterior parieto-occipital region is especially susceptible to watershed infarction. Patients present with hemiplegia or diplegia; the asymmetry is probably due to subtle differences in the vascular supply to the two hemispheres.

*Focal infarcts and trauma:* Focal infarcts and trauma cause typical localizing features referable to the frontal and parietal lobes. The cause is not known in most patients, but focal infarcts may rarely be due to stretching or trauma to the carotid during a difficult delivery.

*Periventricular hemorrhage:* Periventricular hemorrhage occurs in premature infants in the setting of reduced cerebral blood flow (which weakens vessels) being followed by increased blood flow. Hemorrhage develops in periventricular regions; the germinal matrix is especially susceptible.

### Increased Intracranial Pressure
Increased intracranial pressure (ICP) is produced by accumulation of cerebrospinal fluid (CSF), cerebral edema, cerebral mass lesions, and/or extracerebral intracranial mass lesions. Common causes include hydrocephalus, trauma, tumors, hemorrhage, infarction with subsequent edema, and abscess.

Hydrocephalus (discussed below) is accumulation of CSF due to increased production or reduced resorption. Trauma produces contusions, which can have areas of focal cerebral edema. Diffuse cerebral edema after massive cranial trauma is usually devastating. Hemorrhage into the parenchyma of the brain produces focal mass effect; subdural and epidural hematomas produce increased ICP by extrinsic compression of the cerebrum. Subarachnoid hemorrhage increases ICP by a volume effect on the blood and interference with CSF absorption and may produce outflow obstruction from accumulation of blood in the region of the fourth ventricle. Pseudotumor cerebri is increased ICP with no structural lesion found responsible for the increase; the ventricles are not enlarged.

Except for pseudotumor cerebri, increased ICP presents with headache, nausea and vomiting, ataxia, and mental status changes. If the mental status change is profound, the other symptoms may not be apparent. A chronic increase in ICP produces headache and vomiting that are most prominent in the early morning, an unusual pattern for most other causes of headache. If increased ICP is suspected, examination should look for the following findings:

- Papilledema on funduscopic examination is suggestive of increased ICP.
- Cranial nerve palsy and ocular motor palsy can occur with increased ICP in the absence of a focal compressive lesion.
- Cerebellar ataxia and lower cranial neuropathy suggest that a posterior fossa lesion is causing the increased ICP.

Isolated cranial nerve palsy affects cranial nerve (CN) VI most frequently, followed by CN IV and CN III. However, this isolated cranial nerve palsy can be a false localizing finding, since the focal abnormality suggests a locus for a causative lesion that is not found on subsequent diagnostic studies.

Benign intracranial hypertension or pseudotumor cerebri presents with headache but often without other signs of increased ICP. Ocular motor palsies are rare. If untreated, visual loss can occur due to damage to the optic nerve (CN II). Diagnosis requires evaluation for mass lesion and hydrocephalus. Pseudotumur cerebri commonly develops in young obese females.

*Hydrocephalus*
Hydrocephalus is accumulation of CSF and is classified into obstructive hydrocephalus and communicating hydrocephalus.

Obstructive hydrocephalus is due to blockade of ventricular drainage. Locations of blockage include the cerebral aqueduct, interventricular foramen, foramen of Luschka, and foramen of Magendie.

Communicating hydrocephalus is usually due to reduced absorption of CSF from the subarachnoid space, usually because of previous subarachnoid hemorrhage or meningitis. Increased production of CSF can also produce communicating hydrocephalus, commonly from a choroid plexus papilloma.

AQUEDUCT OBSTRUCTION

The aqueduct of Sylvius connects the caudal aspect of the third ventricle with the fourth ventricle. Obstruction of the aqueduct can occur as a result of congenital stenosis, obstruction by midbrain or pineal tumor, intraventricular hemorrhage, or a colloid cyst in the third ventricle. Obstruction produces hydrocephalus affecting the lateral and third ventricles but sparing the fourth.

Patients present with signs of increased ICP, including headache and vomiting, that are most prominent in morning. Associated neurologic symptoms include ataxia of gait and limbs, diplopia, and, if the problem is long-standing, visual change. The ataxia is attributed to damage to axons projecting from the cerebrum to the brain stem and spinal cord. Diplopia may occur because of ocular motor nerve dysfunction or midbrain compression.

Aqueductal obstruction is suspected in patients with signs of increased ICP of subacute or chronic onset. Paroxysmal signs of increased ICP suggest intermittent obstruction, as can occur with colloid cyst of the third ventricle, which produces a ball-valve effect on the aqueduct. Imaging shows increased lateral and third ventricle size with a normal or small fourth ventricle. Magnetic resonance imaging (MRI) may show the exact level of obstruction.

NORMAL PRESSURE HYDROCEPHALUS

Normal pressure hydrocephalus is characterized by increased ventricular size out of proportion to sulcal atrophy. The typical clinical triad is dementia, ataxia, and urinary incontinence, though many patients do not have all three.

Diagnosis is supported by imaging showing ventriculomegaly without prominent sulcal enlargement. Lumbar puncture shows no elevation in pressure. Radionucleotide cisternography shows reflux of isotope in the ventricles. Clinical improvement follows CSF removal.

HYDROCEPHALUS DUE TO MASS LESIONS

Mass lesions may produce hydrocephalus by blocking CSF flow. Occasional tumors may obstruct the interventricular foramen, blocking the flow of CSF from the lateral ventricle to the third ventricle. This barrier produces unilateral hydrocephalus with focal signs referable to the affected hemisphere, including hemiparesis and ataxia. Often patients also have signs of generalized increased ICP. Because of the asymmetric dilation of the lateral ventricle, there may be transcallosal herniation—that is, herniation of cerebral tissue beneath the falx cerebri—following the path of the corpus callosum.

Lesions in the posterior fossa include tumors, hematomas, and abscesses. They can obstruct the drainage of CSF through the foramina of Luschka and Magendie, which produces hydrocephalus affecting the lateral, third, and fourth ventricles. The fourth ventricle may not be visible on computerized tomography (CT) if it is filled with tumor; unfortunately, tumor in the fourth ventricle may be mistaken for normal midline structures on CT. Clues to this diagnosis include all of the signs of cerebral hydrocephalus, plus brain stem findings due to infiltration of the tissue, as well as compression by the enlarged CSF spaces. Headache, ataxia, cranial nerve palsies, and corticospinal tract signs are typical. Diagnosis can be confirmed by MRI. CT often lacks the resolution to visualize posterior fossa structures adequately, but the finding of obstructive hydrocephalus with a fourth ventricle that is enlarged, absent (filled with mass), or deviated to one side is suggestive.

*Encephalitis*

"Encephalitis" means brain inflammation. The most common cause is viral, but nonviral pathogens may also cause encephalitis. Immune-mediated encephalitis is also an important cause.

ACUTE ENCEPHALITIS

Acute encephalitis typically presents with fever, headache, and mental status change. These are nonspecific symptoms, so bacterial meningitis, bacterial cerebritis, tuberculous, and fungal infections must be considered. Mild to moderate CSF pleocytosis supports the diagnosis of acute encephalitis. A markedly elevated CSF white blood cell count suggests a bacterial process. Moderate CSF pleocytosis with high protein levels and very low glucose suggests tuberculous meningitis.

## HERPES SIMPLEX ENCEPHALITIS

Identification of herpes simplex encephalitis is important because treatment with acyclovir has been shown to alter the course of the illness, although most viral encephalitides do not respond to antiviral treatment. Patients can present with all of the symptoms of acute viral encephalitis, including headache, fever, and mental status change. In addition, patients usually have focal signs including hemiparesis, aphasia, visual field deficits, ataxia, cranial nerve palsies, and focal seizures.

There are two subtypes of herpes simplex virus, HSV-1 and HSV-2. HSV-1 causes cold sores, while HSV-2 causes genital herpes. HSV-1 is the most common cause of herpes encephalitis in adults, while HSV-2 is the most common cause in neonates, due to vaginal or transplacental transmission of infection.

HSV encephalitis differs in presentation from most other viral encephalitides because of the predilection for focal damage, especially in the temporal and frontal regions. HSV encephalitis in neonates, however, is global, so focal findings are often absent.

Diagnosis of HSV encephalitis is suspected when a patient with symptoms and signs of encephalitis has focal findings. Diagnosis is supported by imaging and/or EEG showing focal abnormalities, and by CSF pleocytosis; note that the pleocytosis may be polymorphonuclear early in the course. Herpes simplex antibody and antigen testing is routinely available. Brain biopsy is usually not needed; clinical suspicion with supportive laboratory findings provides enough security in the diagnosis to warrant antiviral treatment.

## ARBOVIRUS ENCEPHALITIS

Arboviruses are carried by mosquitoes and ticks. Distinction between individual arboviruses is not clinically important, although it may be important for control of the insect vector. Infection in humans presents as acute encephalitis, with fever, headache, and mental status change.

Differentiation from HSV encephalitis is important, since arbovirus encephalitis does not respond to antiviral therapy. Arbovirus encephalitis lacks the focal findings of and is less fulminant than HSV encephalitis. Overall, the prognosis for full recovery is better with arbovirus encephalitis.

*Developmental Disorders*
Disorders of embryogenesis and neuronal migration can result in a wide spectrum of anatomic anomalies. Most of these present in childhood with developmental delay. Differentiation on clinical grounds is difficult.

Microcephaly refers to a head circumference less than two standard deviations below the mean. Patients with mild microcephaly may be neurologically normal, but severe microcephaly is associated with mental retardation. Primary microcephaly occurs because of a developmental abnormality, whereas secondary microcephaly is due to a disease process that interrupted normal neurological development.

Agenesis of the corpus callosum is the absence or impaired development of the corpus callosum. If the agenesis is partial, the posterior aspect is spared. Agenesis of the corpus callosum is an incidental and asymptomatic finding in many patients. Detailed testing may show defective interhemispheric transfer of information, but this is not clinically important.

Holoprosencephaly is failure of fusion of the forebrain during early development, resulting in a single large ventricle. Corpus callosum is usually absent. Patients present with craniofacial dysplasias such as cleft lip, cleft plate, and cyclopia, often associated with other skeletal malformations.

Defective neuronal migration during early development can result in a reduced number and depth of cortical convolutions (pachygyria), absence of convolutions with a smooth cortical surface (lissencephaly), and abnormal areas of gray matter migration (heterotopia). Patients with defective neuronal migration present with seizures and/or developmental delay. Many patients have dysmorphic features.

*Persistent Vegetative State*

The persistent vegetative state is due to bilateral cerebral dysfunction, with preservation of brain stem function. Common causes include anoxia, bihemispheric infarctions, and head injury, although almost any cause of diffuse cerebral injury can cause this state.

Patients may appear awake but lack normal cerebral reactivity. Brain stem reflexes are intact. Bilateral corticospinal tract damage results in spasticity.

The main differential diagnoses include akinetic mutism, locked-in syndrome, and brain stem causes of coma. Persistent vegetative state is differentiated from akinetic mutism by the corticospinal tract signs and the presence of some primitive spontaneous movements and primitive reactivity; from brain stem destruction by the preservation of brain stem reflexes; and from locked-in syndrome by the absence of both cerebral reactivity and brain stem dysfunction.

*Akinetic Mutism*

Akinetic mutism is the result of bifrontal damage, especially of anterior cingulate gyri, but it may also be due to damage to the midbrain periventricular gray matter, globus pallidus, and/or hypothalamus. Akinetic mutism may develop after hydrocephalus. Patients present with the appearance of being awake but are unresponsive to the environment. The patient's eyes are open but the patient does not follow commands. Pathological reflexes are common, including snout and grasp. Stimulation may produce autonomic reaction but no patterned responsiveness.

Differential diagnoses include brain stem causes of coma and global cerebral dysfunction. Akinetic mutism is sometimes difficult to distinguish from psychogenic unresponsiveness; clues to the latter include inconsistent responsiveness, absence of pathological reflexes, and absence of a probable cause, such as infarction.

*Locked-In Syndrome*

Locked-in syndrome is not characterized by a disturbance in level of consciousness, although coma is often erroneously presumed because of the patient's inability to respond. Locked-in syndrome is discussed further in Chapter 3.

## Multifocal Cerebral Lesions

Multifocal disease is usually diagnosed by history and examination findings suggesting multiple CNS lesions. If the foci are numerous and extensive, differentiation from diffuse processes may be difficult. Important causes of multifocal cerebral pathology include multiple sclerosis, multiple infarctions, abscesses, tumors, and trauma.

Multiple sclerosis affects the white matter. Multiple infarcts from diabetes, atherosclerotic disease, and vasculitis affect both gray and white matter. Some tumors, such as small cell lung cancer and melanoma, have a predilection to multiple metastases.

### Multiple Sclerosis

Multiple sclerosis (MS) is characterized by numerous regions of demyelination with relative preservations of axons. Initial symptoms are due to focal CNS damage and can occur almost anywhere. The most important lesions are of the optic nerve and spinal cord. Patients may present with optic neuritis or transverse myelitis; fortunately, however, only a minority of patients with these isolated conditions develop MS.

Common early symptoms include visual disturbance, hemiparesis or hemisensory loss, myelopathy, dizziness, ataxia, and trigeminal neuralgia. Symptoms may be mild enough to escape attention of patients or physicians for years. When a patient presents with a neurologic deficit that might be MS, the physician must specifically ask about previous neurologic deficits.

The lesions are in the white matter and are easily seen on MRI on T2-weighted images in most patients. Enhanced T1-weighted images may show plaques and may be more sensitive for acute lesions.

Diagnosis is made by findings on history and examination of more than one CNS lesion. MRI may show plaques, but in the absence of clinical findings of multiple lesions, the diagnosis of MS is not made. CSF analysis may show oligoclonal immunoglobulin G (IgG) in the CSF but not in the serum, an abnormal IgG/albumin ratio, myelin basic protein, and/or antibodies to myelin basic protein. None of these findings is diagnostic, and none is 100% specific for MS. However, in the appropriate clinical setting, these CSF abnormalities can support the diagnosis. Evoked potentials (EPs) can provide supportive evidence of MS by showing clinically silent lesions. For example, in a patient with optic neuritis, an abnormal visual evoked potential is expected, but an abnormal somatosensory evoked potential may suggest a spinal or cerebral lesion and, therefore, MS. Diagnostic categories include the following:

- Clinically definite MS
- Laboratory-supported definite MS
- Clinically probable MS
- Laboratory-supported probable MS

Diagnosis of clinically definite MS requires two attacks and clinical signs of two separate neurologic lesions. Laboratory-supported definite MS requires two attacks and clinical signs of one lesion plus MRI or EP evidence of an addition lesion, or a single attack with associated clinical findings plus clinical or MRI or EP evidence of another lesion. Laboratory evidence includes oligoclonal bands or increased IgG in the CSF.

A diagnosis of clinically probable MS requires two attacks with clinical signs of one lesion, or one attack with associated clinical findings with clinical, MRI, or EP evidence of another lesion. Laboratory-supported probable MS requires two attacks with CSF abnormalities, as above.

In the clinical evaluation of a patient, the examiner should consider whether all of the patient's symptoms can be explained by one lesion; if not, then multifocal disorders such as MS should be considered.

*Multiple Infarctions*
Multiple cerebral infarctions can develop in patients with advanced atherosclerotic disease, diabetes mellitus, CNS vasculitis, and systemic lupus erythematosus (SLE) and cardiac emboli.

CNS vasculitis may be isolated or a component of a systemic vasculitis. Patients often present with headache and varied neurologic findings, including ataxia, hemiparesis, hemisensory loss, visual obscuration, and nonspecific dizziness.

SLE commonly produces neurologic symptoms. In addition to CNS dysfunction, there may be peripheral nervous system dysfunction as well; some patients develop significant neuropathy. Trigeminal neuropathy can develop; the location of the lesion is probably at the trigeminal ganglion.

Antiphospholipid antibody syndrome is characterized by multiple cerebral infarctions, which affect the white and gray matter. Clinically, the infarctions are indistinguishable from those due to multiple proximal emboli, and this diagnosis needs to be excluded. Laboratory findings may include positive antinuclear antibody, thrombocytopenia, false-positive VDRL results, and an abnormal Russell's viper venom time. Hemorrhage can occur, but infarctions are much more common. Antiphospholipid antibodies are responsible for only a small proportion of strokes in young adults but may be present in 30 to 40 percent of patients with SLE.

*Abscesses and Tumors*
Abscesses can be single or multiple; when multiple, they present with multifocal signs and symptoms. Brain abscesses develop due to extension of infection from structures near the brain or from hematogenous dissemination. Spread of infection from the mastoid or other sinuses usually produces solitary abscesses. Hematogenous dissemination has a predilection for multiple abscesses. Multiple abscesses are prevalent with subacute bacterial endocarditis, acquired immunodeficiency syndrome, congenital heart disease, and lung abscesses. The examiner needs to consider nonneurologic involvement, proximal emboli, and immune deficiency. Evaluation may include echocardiogram, blood cultures, urine culture, complete blood count, human immunodeficiency virus test, and chest x-ray.

Tumors that have a predilection to multiple metastases include small cell lung cancer, breast cancer, melanoma, and gastrointestinal tumors. In a patient with known cancer, multifocal signs and symptoms should be clues to possible multiple metastases. This possibility is especially a concern in older patients with recent-onset focal seizures. Contrasted CT can show metastases, but MRI is clearly superior.

*Trauma*

Trauma commonly produces multiple areas of cerebral dysfunction. The frontal and temporal poles are especially prone to damage. Damage occurs with sudden acceleration and deceleration of the brain, as in a car accident. Contusion may occur in areas of direct tissue injury under the point of impact (coup injury) and in areas of recoil injury opposite the point of impact (contrecoup injury).

Most patients with contusions suffered loss of consciousness at the time of injury. Most patients do not have hemorrhages, but bleeding into the site of a contusion or epidural or subdural hematoma can occur late in a few patients.

Mild head injury is often associated with headache, dizziness, and nausea. More severe injury results in lethargy or coma. Focal neurologic signs suggest parenchymal hematoma. Subdural and epidural hematomas may produce focal signs but more often result in signs of increased ICP.

CT is indicated in patients with significant head injury, especially in the presence of focal signs or alteration of consciousness. Imaging is not needed if the patient has no complaints and is neurologically intact, although the patient and family should be warned to watch for late signs of hemorrhage. Plain radiographs are not sufficient for evaluation of significant head injury.

### Focal Cerebral Lesions

Focal lesions have many possible etiologies. While tumors and missile injuries can affect almost any location, infarctions follow vascular distributions. Figure 1.4 shows the vascular supply of the cerebral cortex. Subcortical circulation is discussed below by structure. Table 1.2 lists the clinical findings with common cerebral vascular syndromes.

*Frontal Lobe Lesions*

Symptoms and signs produced by lesion of the frontal lobes include the following:

- Akinesia
- Apraxia
- Paratonia
- Frontal lobe ataxia
- Behavioral change
- Frontal release signs

Akinesia is a tendency not to use the affected extremity despite preserved muscle power. Akinesia of frontal origin is often confused with parkinsonism.

Apraxia is a defect in performing a sequence of movements despite the ability to perform each component of the task.

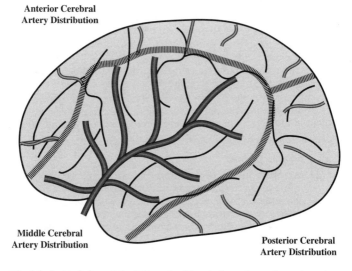

**Anterior Cerebral Artery Distribution**

**Middle Cerebral Artery Distribution**

**Posterior Cerebral Artery Distribution**

**Fig. 1.4** Lateral view of the left cerebral hemisphere shows the major arteries supplying the cortex.

**Table 1.2   Vascular Syndromes**

| Vessel | Involved Structures | Findings |
|---|---|---|
| **Infarction** | | |
| Anterior cerebral artery | Parasagittal cortex, especially frontal lobe | Contralateral leg weakness and sensory loss, with a lesser degree of proximal arm deficits; sphincter dysfunction, contralateral frontal release signs, paratonia |
| MCA: superior division | Broca's area, primary motor and sensory cortices | Contralateral hemiparesis, hemisensory loss; if dominant hemisphere, Broca's aphasia |
| MCA: inferior division | Wernicke's area, optic radiations | Wernicke's aphasia: hemianopia or superior quadrantanopia |
| MCA: both divsons | All of the above | All of the above |
| PCA | Occipital cortex, rostral midbrain, inferior portion of internal capsule, medial temporal lobe | Contralateral hemianopia, memory deficits with inferior temporal involvement; if bilateral, cortical blindness |
| Lenticulostriate arteries, branches of MCA | Internal capsule, basal ganglia | Pure motor hemiplegia; possible extrapyramidal symptoms with basal ganglia involvement |
| Thalamoperforate arteries, branches of PCA | Thalamus, inferior, medial, and anterior aspects | Contralateral sensory loss, thlamic pain syndrome; possible movement disorder, including hemiballismus and choreoathetosis |

**Table 1.2** *(continued)*

| Vessel | Involved Structures | Findings |
| --- | --- | --- |
| Internal carotid artery | MCA artery distribution; possible ACA involvement as well | Hemiplegia, hemisensory loss, aphasia with dominant hemisphere lesions; possible headache |
| *Venous Thrombosis* | | |
| Superior sagittal sinous thrombosis | Venous drainage from the hemispheres and medial cerebral cortex | Increased intracranial pressure, headache, bilateral corticospinal tract signs, encephalopathy, high mortality |
| Transverse sinus thrombosis | Venous drainage from the posterior fossa, as well as drainage from the confluence of sinuses | Pain, especially behind the ear; Increased intracranial pressure |
| Cavernous sinus thrombosis | Cranial nerves IV, V, and/or VI; internal carotid artery, possible ophthalmic artery | Retro-orbital pain, proptosis, orbital congestion; possible facial sensory loss, signs of carotid artery occlusion; visual loss |
| *Hemorrhage* | | |
| Cerebral lobe | Respective cerebral lobe, often with mass effect distorting neighboring structures | Acute-onset headache, neurologic deficit, nausea with or without vomiting; stupor or coma with increased intracranial pressure |
| Basal ganglia | Putamen especially | Headache, contralateral hemiparesis, nausea with or without vomiting |

**Table 1.2** *(continued)*

| Vessel | Involved Structures | Findings |
| --- | --- | --- |
| Pons | Pons, including ascending and descending tracts, cranial nerves | Sudden-onset coma, quadriparesis; loss of brain stem reflexes, including doll's-head |
| Cerebellum | Cerebellar hemisphere with compression of other brain stem structures | Occipital headache, vomiting, gait ataxia; possible ipsilateral facial weakness and decreased corneal reflex |
| Subdural | Venous blood, hematoma layered over the convexity; often bilateral, with mixed acute and chronic blood | *Acute:* encephalopathy or loss of consciousness without a lucid interval; *Chronic:* encephalopathy, possible headache, few focal signs |
| Epidural | Usually arterial blood; hematoma in a lens shape impinging on the cortex | Frequent early loss of consciousness followed by awakening; later onset of headache, vomiting, drowsiness, hemiparesis, seizures |

MCA = middle cerebral artery; PCA = posterior cerebral artery; ACA = anterior cerebral artery.

Paratonia is a state of increased tone with passive movement that tends to oppose the imparted movement; nevertheless, the patient with paratonia can move the extremity well. The examiner often initially believes that the patient is not being cooperative. A catch in the muscle with initiation of movement might suggest the cogwheel rigidity of parkinsonism, but it feels different, being irregular and lacking the rhythmic catch–release of parkinsonism.

Frontal lobe ataxia is characterized by difficulty initiating gait (feet seem stuck to the floor), short and shuffling steps on a narrow base, and difficulty turning. As with akinesia, frontal lobe ataxia is often confused with parkinsonism, but it is differentiated by the presence of frontal release signs and the absence of other signs of parkinsonism, such as tremor.

Behavioral changes with frontal lobe lesions include mood changes, emotional volatility, and attention difficulties. Table 1.3 lists some of the mood alterations common with frontal lobe lesions. Frontal release signs are pathological reflexes and include the following types:

- Grasp
- Palmomental
- Snout
- Suck
- Glabellar

None of these frontal release signs are normally present in healthy adults, and their presence suggests a contralateral frontal lobe lesion. However, these findings are not always specific to frontal lobe damage and may be seen in diffuse disorders, including AD.

**Table 1.3   Behavioral Changes with Frontal Lobe Lesions**

| Behavior | Lesion Location |
| --- | --- |
| Depression; may include pathological crying | Left frontal lobe; possible extensive subcortical lesions, especially bilaterally |
| Inappropriate cheerfulness; may include pathological laughter | Right frontal lobe |
| Flat affect; apathy | Bilateral medial–frontal or bilateral anterior temporal–temporal lobes |
| Aprosodic speech (lack of emotional intonation) | Right frontal lobe |
| Akinetic mutism | Bilateral medial frontal lobe, midbrain periventricular gray matter, or hydrocephalus |

The examiner elicits the grasp reflex by gently stroking the palm of the patient's hand with his or her fingers. A mildly positive response is hooking of the fingers; a marked grasp is forced closure of the hand around the examiner's fingers despite specific instructions not to hold on to the hand. Damage to the medial aspect of the premotor cortex (area 6) produces a grasp response. I have found the grasp to be the most reliable pathological reflex indicating frontal lobe dysfunction.

The palmomental reflex is elicited by stroking the palm of the hand more briskly than for the grasp; I use the back side of my fingernail. A positive response is contraction of the mentalis, producing slight depression of the lower lip, ipsilateral to the side being stimulated. Lesion of the frontal lobe produces the palmomental reflex; precise localization is not possible.

The snout reflex is elicited by lightly tapping the upper lip. A snout is pursing of the lips. In severe cases, the lips may purse with approach of an object even without contact; such a response is, strictly speaking, the rooting reflex, but it has the same clinical implications.

Closing of the mouth around an object is the suck reflex, and it is easily elicited by use of a tongue depressor. Stroking the tongue depressor on the side of the mouth facilitates the reflex.

The glabellar reflex is also know as the blink reflex. It is elicited by tapping over the supraorbital ridge and observing reflex contraction of the orbicularis oculi. With frontal lobe lesions and Parkinson's disease, patients are often not able to suppress the reflex.

Important causes of frontal lobe lesions include the following:

- Tumors
- Infarctions
- Head injuries

Relevant tumors include olfactory groove meningiomas, unilateral frontal lobe tumors, butterfly gliomas, and parasagittal tumors. Olfactory groove meningiomas produce damage to the inferior frontal region, with resultant personality and intellectual changes but few other signs; unfortunately, smell is not commonly tested in clinical practice. Unilateral frontal lobe tumors produce frontal release signs contralateral to the lesion; they usually produces less personality change than bilateral involvement does. Butterfly gliomas received their name because they infiltrate the white matter of the frontal lobes and cross through the anterior aspect of the corpus callosum, giving a butterfly appearance on enhanced CT or MRI. These tumors produce intellectual and behavioral changes, often associated with signs of increased ICP, including headache, nausea with or without vomiting, and papilledema. Parasagittal tumors are usually meningiomas, and they usually present with intellectual disturbances, behavioral changes (especially apathy), and incontinence; the incontinence should be a clue that the patient's problem is not purely psychiatric.

Infarctions of the frontal lobe are due to anterior cerebral artery occlusion, which produces all of the same symptoms seen with other midline frontal lesions, except that the onset is sudden rather than insidious. Anterior cerebral artery occlusion can cause bilateral medial frontal infarction when both the left and right anterior cerebral arteries arise from the same trunk.

Head trauma produces damage, especially to the frontal and temporal poles. Damage to the frontal lobes through initial injury or subsequent edema commonly produces behavioral and intellectual disturbances, which are often of tremendous concern to families. Social inhibitions may be lost, resulting in inappropriate sexual behavior, impulsivity, and errors in judgment. Intellectual powers do not always change in parallel with the behavioral alteration, and there are many examples of patients who have substantial personality change yet still excel at school or work.

### Parietal Lobe Lesions

Parietal lesions affect mainly sensory function and sensorimotor integration. The most anterior aspect of the parietal lobe is the sensory strip, on the postcentral gyrus; lesion here produces sensory loss in a region appropriate to the sensory homunculus. The inferior parietal region includes the supramarginal gyrus and angular gyrus; lesion of the supramarginal gyrus affects speech, and lesion of the angular gyrus affects speech and reading, as described earlier in this chapter.

The sensory deficit with cerebral cortical lesions is termed "cortical sensory loss," which means that the patient may be able to identify primitive sensory modalities but has difficulty synthesizing the sensory information into meaningful concepts. For example, the patient may have difficulty identifying of coins in his or her hand (astereognosis) or recognizing numbers written in the palm of the hand (dysgraphesthesia).

Parietal lesions confined to the cortex do not directly alter visual fields, but many lesions affecting the parietal cortex affect the optic radiations in the underlying white matter, producing an incomplete hemianopia that affects the inferior quadrant.

The form of apraxia seen differs with parietal lobe lesions in the dominant and nondominant hemispheres. Patients with dominant hemisphere lesions in the inferior parietal lobe have ideomotor apraxia and have more difficulty using the hand to mimic tasks than actually performing the task with a tool; such patients often use the hand as the tool. For example, when asked to imitate the use of a hammer, the patient may make a fist and swing it as the hammer head, rather that make the motion of grasping a hammer handle. This apraxia can also occur with frontal lesions, however. Apraxia with aphasia would suggest a dominant hemisphere lesion; apraxia without aphasia would suggest a nondominant hemisphere lesion. Apraxia is discussed further later in this chapter.

Gerstmann's syndrome is due to a lesion in the angular gyrus. The quartet of clinical features includes agraphia, right–left disorientation, acalculia, and finger agnosia. Patients often have anomia and alexia, the latter due to damage to associative interactions between visual processing areas and language centers.

Conduction aphasia is the inability to repeat a spoken word or phrase. Spontaneous speech may be preserved, so there is a marked discrepancy between conversation and repetition. Often, however, some expressive problems and anomia are also present, but to a lesser extent than the difficulty with repetition.

*Temporal Lobe Lesions*

The temporal lobes are concerned with multiple functions, most of which integrate sensory and motor modalities. The medial temporal lobe, including the hippocampus, is important for memory.

Pure word deafness is due to unilateral or bilateral lesions separating Wernicke's area from Heschl's gyri; the separation is often due to white matter lesion(s). The salient feature is severely impaired auditory reception with relative preservation of reading, writing, and speaking. Reading is preserved because the visual input is not processed at the primary auditory cortex but, rather, is associated with language functions in the parietal lobe. Pure word deafness is uncommon and may be missed if not expressly looked for; a patient with posterior aphasia may surprise the examiner or family by demonstrating the ability to read.

Damage to the temporal lobes may result in behavioral disturbances, including mood disorders, alterations in sexual behavior, and elements of the "temporal lobe personality" already discussed. Damage to the anterior and medial aspects especially predisposes to abnormalities; this damage can occur in head injuries with temporal contusion, herpes simplex encephalitis, and neoplasms affecting this area.

Memory disorders can occur with temporal lobe lesions, especially if the damage is bilateral. Memories are probably not directly stored in the temporal lobes, since resection of one or the other temporal lobe does not abolish selected memories. Damage to one temporal lobe can result in a memory deficit, but this is usually transient. The Wada test is often performed before surgical ablation of a temporal lobe to remove an epileptic focus or tumor; this test helps to predict the effect of surgery on language and memory. Damage to the left temporal lobe produces deficits in verbal memory while damage to the right temporal lobe affects nonverbal memory.

Meyer's loop is an arc of axons that is part of the optic radiations. The loop extends through the white matter of the temporal lobe. Damage to the temporal lobe affecting these axons produces a defect in the contralateral superior quadrant of the visual field.

*Occipital Lobe Lesions*

Symptoms and signs of occipital lobe lesions are predominantly visual; they are discussed in the section on visual abnormalities. Table 1.8 (below) summarizes the effects of lesions on vision.

An occipital lobe lesion is suggested by visual field abnormalities that are similar for both eyes. Differentiation among optic tract, optic radiation, and occipital lobe lesions is difficult on clinical grounds; associated nonvisual symptoms are useful.

*Parasagittal Lesions*

A parasagittal frontal lesion may produce gait difficulty characterized by small shuffling steps; this finding may be confused with parkinsonism. The gait difficulty is not explained by the degree of leg spasticity, which may be the result of concurrent corticospinal tract dysfunction.

Parasagittal lesions in the frontocentral region can produce incontinence and bilateral leg weakness, which may be erroneously attributed to a spinal cord lesion. A parasagittal lesion may be differentiated from a cord lesion by the absence of back pain and the presence of cerebral symptoms (including memory difficulty), behavioral changes (including apathy), and occasionally headache. Differentiation on a clinical basis is occasionally impossible; if a patient presents with symptoms and signs of myelopathy but evaluation is unrevealing, a parasagittal lesion must be considered.

Parasagittal lesions in the occipital region can produce cortical blindness.

## MOTOR AND SENSORY DYSFUNCTION

### Weakness

Weakness of cortical origin follows the topographical organization of the motor strip (Figure 1.3). Since vascular lesions predominate, vascular anatomy guides the symptoms that develop. Infarction of the superior division of the middle cerebral artery affects the lateral aspect of the precentral gyrus, which controls face and arm movement; leg movement may be affected due to infarction of the white fiber tracts descending from the medial aspect of the precentral cortex. Infarction in an anterior cerebral distribution affects the medial aspect of the precentral gyrus, producing leg weakness. The weakness affects distal muscles predominantly, especially foot dorsiflexors and intrinsic muscles of the foot. Bilateral involvement may occur because of the proximity of the medial frontal regions; bilateral leg weakness and spasticity can be confused with a myelopathy.

**Sensory Loss**

Sensory loss can obviously occur with lesions at any level of the neuraxis, and the key to localizing the lesion is defining the sensory loss. Unfortunately, sensory examination is often confusing, and the results may seem nonanatomical. This confusion does not mean that the patient has functional sensory loss; instead, the patient may be trying to help the examiner, whether consciously or uncon-

**Table 1.4   General Guide to Sensory Loss**

| Level of Lesion | Features and Location of Sensory Loss |
|---|---|
| Cortical | Contralateral body; loss restricted to a portion of the homunculus; if the entire side is affected, one limb is affected more than others; weakness common |
| Internal capsule | Contralateral body; loss often involves the face, arm, and leg equally; weakness common; sensory loss without weakness highly suggestive |
| Thalamus | Contralateral body; loss usually involves face, arm, leg, and trunk; may seem to split the midline |
| Spinal transection | Sensory loss at and below a segmental level; which may seem slightly different for each side |
| Spinal hemisection | Sensory loss ipsilateral for vibration and proprioception (dorsal columns), contralateral for pain and temperature (spinothalamic tracts) |
| Nerve root | Follows dermatomal distribution (see Chapter 5) |
| Plexus | May span two or more adjacent dermatomal distributions, especially C5–6, C8–T1, and L5–S1 |
| Peripheral nerve | Follows peripheral nerve anatomy (see Chapter 5) |

sciously. Variability between individuals in sensory distribution is another consideration.

Table 1.4 is a guide to differentiation of sensory deficits at different levels of the neuraxis. Only cortical and cerebral subcortical sensory syndromes are discussed in this section; see related chapters for sensory losses related to brain stem, spinal, and peripheral nerve lesions.

Cortical sensory loss is differentiated from subcortical lesions because the loss follows the topographic organization of the sensory strip. Also, a cortical lesion is unlikely to produce sensory loss without motor loss, due to the proximity of the motor and sensory strips.

Cortical sensory loss crosses boundaries of innervation made up by single nerves, roots, and spinal levels. The hand and face are prominently represented on the cortex, so they are strongly affected by cortical lesions. Distal aspects of the hand are more affected than proximal aspects. The most common cortical sensory loss in clinical practice is due to infarction; sensory loss from cortical infarction can be from lesions of the middle cerebral, anterior cerebral, or penetrating arteries. Table 1.5 shows features of the sensory loss associated with each of these.

### Apraxia

Apraxia is a disorder of movement not due to loss of strength, abnormal tone, or defect in the error-correction mechanisms of the body. To determine that a patient has apraxia, the examiner must believe that the patient understands the task; the defect is in execution of the concept. For example, a patient may be able to manipulate a screwdriver and may even be able to indicate an awareness of the association with a screw, but he or she is unable to place the blade in the slot and turn the screw. The various forms of apraxia are enumerated below.

The prototypic apraxia is ideomotor. Apraxia for sequential tasks and apraxia for objects used to be subsumed under the title "ideational apraxia." Limb-kinetic apraxia is an impairment in fine coordination without weakness; it is due to mild corticospinal tract

**Table 1.5 Sensory Loss Associated with Vascular Lesions**

| Vessel | Region Infarcted | Clinical Features |
|--------|------------------|-------------------|
| Anterior cerebral artery | Medial aspect of central region adjacent to sagittal sinus | Contralateral leg; arm and face usually spared; most prominent distally |
| Middle cerebral artery | Lateral aspect of fronto-parietal cortex | Contralateral arm and face; leg spared; most prominent distally |
| Lenticulostriate artery | Internal capsule | Contralateral body; each region affected almost equally; little or no motor loss |
| Thalamoperforate artery | Thalamus | Contralateral body; each region affected almost equally; little or no motor loss; possible thalmic pain syndrome |

dysfunction rather than being a true apraxia, and it is not discussed here.

### *Ideomotor Apraxia*

Ideomotor apraxia is impairment in the ability to perform a motor task while being able to understand the command and having the required motor skills to perform the task. This condition is what most clinicians look for when they test for apraxia. The deficit is prominent with pantomime and less so when the patient uses the real object.

The lesions producing ideomotor apraxia are generally confined to the left hemisphere, and associated symptoms depend on the location of the lesion. The normal pathway for carrying out a verbal command begins with auditory decoding of the command in Wernicke's area, relay of the command to the left premotor area via the arcuate fasciculus, and relay of the individual motor commands to the left motor cortex for right limb movement. If the left limb is to carry out the command, the information is relayed from the left premotor area to the right premotor area via the corpus callosum. The motor commands are then relayed to the right motor cortex for execution of the task.

The most common cause of ideomotor apraxia is a lesion of the left frontal lobe that has damaged the premotor area directly. The right arm may be too weak to be testable, but apraxia of the left is obvious if tested for. Many patients will have anterior aphasia but still be able to understand the task. Midline frontal lesions can interrupt the connection between premotor areas without affecting them directly; in this case, use of the right arm is unimpaired, but apraxia with the left arm is evident. Lesions of the parietal and posterior temporal regions are said to produce ideomotor apraxia, but it is not clear that the patients understand the task and/or recognize the correct performance of the task. Patients with parietal lesions affecting the arcuate fasciculus seldom have right hemiparesis, though they do have conduction aphasia. Patients with a lesion in Wernicke's area have been shown to exhibit ideomotor apraxia by their inability to perform skilled tasks demonstrated by the examiner, but the interpretation of these data is controversial.

### Apraxia for Sequential Tasks

With apraxia for sequential tasks, there is impaired performance of a complex multistep task. The classic example is lighting a pipe, from filling the bowl to lighting to smoking. Lesions are usually in the frontal lobe, affecting centers involved in sequential motor planning. The lesions may not be focal but diffuse, as in AD and other dementing illnesses.

### Apraxia for Objects

With apraxia for objects, the patient cannot use real objects for their intended use. This condition affects activities of daily living, including brushing teeth, shaving, and bathing. The symptoms can be seen with focal lesions, but they are much more common in diffuse disorders, such as AD and other dementing illnesses.

## Constructional Apraxia

To test for constructional apraxia, the patient is asked to copy drawings such as a three-dimensional box or house. A common task is to draw a circle, then fill in the numbers as if it were the face of a clock. An affected patient will make errors in perspective and assembly. For the diagnosis to be made, the patient must understand the task and must be physically able to make the required movements with the hand. Classically, constructional apraxia is due to right hemisphere damage, although patients with constructional difficulty due to left hemisphere lesions have been described. It is believed that constructional apraxia is caused by a deficit in visuospatial integration during performance of motor tasks, implicating the parietal region. Severely affected patients may copy geometric designs as unrecognizable representations of the original. Patients may fill in the numbers of the clock only on one side of the face, indicating neglect of one hemifield.

## Akinesia

Akinesia is commonly thought of as a sign of extrapyramidal dysfunction, but it can also be seen with lesions of the medial frontal lobes; the contralateral limbs retain strength, though there is a tendency to not use them for tasks. The gait is often confused with parkinsonism; there is difficulty initiating movement, short and shuffling steps, and impaired turning. Bilateral frontal lobe dysfunction is unusual with purely cortical lesions; rather, it is seen with lesions such as infarctions, demyelinating diseases, tumors such as butterfly gliomas and bifrontal metastases, and hydrocephalus.

Abnormalities of tone frequently accompany akinesia from frontal lesions. Lesion of the premotor cortex (area 6) produces paratonia—that is, tone develops in a limb, and passive movement tends to oppose the imparted movement, yet the patient can make the same movements voluntarily. It often seems that the patient is simply not cooperating with instructions to relax for passive movement.

## APHASIA

Aphasia is an acquired disorder of language secondary to brain
damage. Aphasia must be distinguished from motor disorders of
speech, such as dysarthria and dysphonia, which affect speech but
not the central processes of language. Also, aphasia must be distinguished from thought disorders that affect language content without a direct effect on language function, such as schizophrenia.
Table 1.6 summarizes language disorders and associated lesions.
Table 1.7 is a guide to clinical differentiation of the disorders.

**Table 1.6  Language Disorders**

| Disorder | Features | Lesion |
|---|---|---|
| Anomia | Impaired naming | Left hemisphere |
| Anterior aphasia | Expressive difficulty with preserved comprehension | Posterior aspect of left inferior frontal lobule; Broca's area |
| Posterior aphasia | Poor comprehension; speech sounds fluent but devoid of content | Left superior temporal gyrus; Wernicke's area |
| Alexia without agraphia | Inability to read with preserved writing | Interruption of the fibers from both occipital lobes to the dominant temporo-parietal region; possible single lesion in the white matter near the occipital horn of the lateral ventricle |
| Aphemia | Impaired speech without impaired writing | Small lesion in Broca's area or subcortical white matter |
| Transcortical motor aphasia | Expressive difficulty with preserved repetition | Inferior frontal lobe anterior to Broca's area |
| Transcortical sensory aphasia | Difficulty with comprehension but preserved repetition | Posterior temporal–occipital region, posterior to Wernicke's area |

**Table 1.7   Clinical Differentiation of Language Disorders**

| Aphasia Type | Fluency | Comprehension | Repetition |
|---|---|---|---|
| Broca's or anterior | Poor | Adequate | Poor |
| Wernicke's or posterior | Adequate | Poor | Poor |
| Conduction | Adequate | Adequate | Poor |
| Global | Poor | Poor | Poor |
| Transcortical motor | Poor | Adequate | Adequate |
| Transcortical sensory | Adequate | Poor | Adequate |
| Transcortical global | Poor | Poor | Adequate |

Adapted from Damasio, NEJM 326:532-9, 1992.

### Anterior Aphasia

Anterior aphasia is also called Broca's aphasia. Minimally, a lesion of Broca's area on the inferior frontal gyrus is required for diagnosis, though larger lesions are often present. Clinical features include hesitant or telegraphic speech. In severe cases the patient may be mute, unable to communicate verbally or in writing. When the patient can speak, anomia and difficulty with repetition, reading aloud, and writing are common, despite relatively preserved comprehension. Patients are aware of their deficit and frustrated; they know what they want to say but have difficulty getting it out. Often, they will have difficulty with a particular word or phrase and will talk around the subject. Most patients have some hemiparesis, though not all; when hemiparesis is present, the face and arm are affected more than the leg. This finding is probably due to the most common cause of anterior aphasia, infarction in the distribution of the anterior division of the middle cerebral artery. Depression is common, probably due to the patient's frustration with the deficit.

### Posterior Aphasia

Posterior aphasia is also called Wernicke's aphasia. Lesion of the superior temporal region is required for the diagnosis, although larger lesions are often present, frequently extending into the parietal lobe. Clinical features include receptive difficulty with relative preservation of speech. The patients are often unaware of their errors in expression, so their speech is devoid of meaning while filled with common words and phrases and punctuated with inflections. Paraphrasic errors are typical, and a patient may be quite convinced of the accuracy of an errant name. Reading may be preserved with restricted lesions, but this is uncommon.

Because of the location of the lesions, hemiparesis is uncommon. In contrast to patients with anterior aphasia, patients are seldom depressed. Because they are often unaware of their deficit, speech therapy is difficult.

### Global Aphasia

Global aphasia is the sum of anterior and posterior aphasias, and it is usually due to extensive infarction in the distribution of the middle cerebral artery. Because of the size of the lesion, hemiparesis, hemisensory loss, and hemianopia are common.

### Anomia

Anomia is impairment of naming; it is common with left hemisphere lesions and cannot be localized to one isolated region of the cortex. Anomia occurs with many lesions, whether focal or diffuse. For example, anomia can occur with parietal, temporal, and frontal lesions and with diffuse disorders, such as AD and anoxia.

### Transcortical Aphasias

Transcortical aphasias are due to disconnection of language centers from other cortical regions. The key to these disorders is preservation of repetition, indicating that the primary receptive and expressive centers are intact, including their interconnections.

Transcortical motor aphasia is characterized by expressive difficulty, similar to that seen with anterior aphasia, and by preservation of repetition and comprehension. The lesion is anterior to Broca's area on the frontal lobe.

Transcortical sensory aphasia is characterized by difficulty with comprehension, similar to that seen with posterior aphasia, and by relative preservation of expression and repetition. The lesion is in the left posterior temporo-occipital region, posterior to the primary auditory cortex and Wernicke's area.

Transcortical global aphasia has features of both anterior and posterior aphasias with preservation of repetition; this aphasia is quite rare. Transcortical global aphasia is usually due to large watershed infarction of the left hemisphere.

Thalamic infarction in the dominant hemisphere can result in an aphasia that has the clinical appearance of a transcortical aphasia. Infarctions in the basal ganglia have also been described as causing aphasia.

### Conduction Aphasia

Conduction aphasia is the inability to repeat a spoken word or phrases. Spontaneous speech may be well-preserved, and there is a marked discrepancy between conversation and repetition. Often, however, some expressive problems and anomia are also present, but to a lesser extent than the difficulty with repetition. Conduction aphasia can be produced by lesions of the superior temporal or inferior parietal regions; lesion of the arcuate fasciculus is thought by many to be important, although this is controversial.

### DEMENTIA

Dementia is a decline in intellectual function. A chronic process is usually implied, while more acute and subacute disorders are called "encephalopathies," a less specific term. Dementia is divided into two major categories: cortical and subcortical.

Cortical dementia is predominantly due to degeneration of neurons in the cerebral cortex, although degeneration in other areas also occurs. Patients present with prominent cortical symptoms, including aphasia, apraxia, and agnosia. Subcortical functions such as gait and coordination are preserved. The preservation of gait, along with dysfunction of higher cortical functions, results in the typical wandering behavior of patients with cortical dementias; this is an important differentiating feature from subcortical dementias.

Subcortical dementia is due to dysfunction of deep nuclei and/or the axons comprising cortical–subcortical and cortical–cortical associative connections. Patients present with intellectual dysfunction although cortical functions are relatively preserved. Gait is often prominently affected.

**Cortical Dementias**

The most important cortical dementias are AD and Pick's disease. Clinical clues can guide differentiation, but pathology is required for definitive diagnosis. Diffuse Lewy body disease is being increasingly recognized.

*Alzheimer's Disease*

Alzheimer's disease is characterized by widespread degeneration of neurons in the brain, with a prominent loss of cholinergic neurons projecting from the nucleus basalis to the cortex. Patients present with memory loss and various combinations of aphasia, apraxia, agnosia, and visuospatial disturbance. Late in the course, gait, continence, and social skills are affected. Behavioral changes may include depression, agitation, withdrawal, delusions, paranoia, and sometimes hallucinations.

AD is differentiated from other dementias by history and examination findings and by laboratory tests to evaluate for other causes. Useful differentiating features include the following:

- Rate of progression
- Aphasia
- Gait
- Absence of focal neurologic signs

AD progresses over years in a slow and steady process. This pattern is helpful in differentiating AD from vascular dementia, which usually shows a stepwise pattern. Some patients with AD may seem to have acute onset or exacerbation, especially after an injury or surgical procedure, but careful history usually elicits symptoms prior to the event.

Aphasia is common in the early stages of AD. Patients have difficulty naming things and often use word substitutions and make paraphrasic errors. Articulation and comprehension are preserved until later stages of the disease. Aphasia may suggest a focal dominant hemisphere lesion, but in the absence of other signs of focal cerebral dysfunction, such as weakness, incoordination, and reflex asymmetry, some elements of aphasia are common in AD.

Gait is relatively preserved in mild to moderate AD, resulting in wandering behavior. Many other causes of dementia are associated with abnormalities in gait and posture, including hydrocephalus, vascular dementia, and diffuse Lewy body disease.

Focal neurologic signs are rarely seen in AD; if present, focal signs would suggest a structural abnormality, such as brain tumor or stroke.

### Pick's Disease

Pick's disease is difficult to differentiate from AD on clinical grounds. Patients with Pick's disease are reported to have more frontal lobe findings (including apathy) than patients with AD, gait difficulty from frontal lobe dysfunction, and more prominent dysphasia early in the course of the disease. Otherwise, patients present with slowly progressive dementia without focal signs. The frontal lobe gait disturbance is characterized by a narrow-based gait with shuffling features, which can be mistaken for parkinsonism.

Premortem diagnosis is by suspicion. Positron emission tomography may show prominent hypometabolism in a frontal–temporal distribution.

### Diffuse Lewy Body Disease

Diffuse Lewy body disease is characterized by dementia plus parkinsonism features, including rigidity and bradykinesia. Pathology shows Lewy bodies distributed widely in the cerebral cortex plus changes more typical of AD. Diagnosis is confirmed only at autopsy, but it is suggested by the finding of dementia early in the course of the parkinsonism. Is should be noted, however, that patients with moderate to advanced AD commonly have rigidity and bradykinesia.

## Subcortical Dementias

Subcortical dementias are differentiated from cortical dementias by relative sparing of speech and praxis. Common causes of subcortical dementia are vascular diseases, MS, and degenerative diseases that predominantly affect white matter and deep nuclei.

### Vascular Dementia

Vascular dementia is also know as multi-infarct dementia (MID). It is believed that 10 to 25 percent of demented patients have MID. The keys to diagnosis include the following:

- Multifocal signs on neurologic examination
- Stepwise progression of the deficit
- Cardiovascular risk factors or a history of significant cardiovascular or cerebrovascular disease

Not all of these findings will invariably be present, but the absence of one or more is strong evidence against vascular dementia, regardless of the findings on CT and/or MRI. Care is needed when interpreting MRI findings in the elderly, since most elderly patients will have white matter changes that are not significant.

### Multiple Sclerosis

MS is often associated with cognitive changes, which may predate the clinical diagnosis. Early signs of dementia due to MS may initially be attributed to affective disturbances.

### Parkinson's Disease

Estimates of the incidence of dementia in Parkinson's disease (PD) differ widely, but 30 percent is a good compromise. There is also disagreement about the pathophysiology of the dementia; some researchers believe that it is the result of AD coinciding with PD, and others claim that it is the result of other biochemical alterations. The occurrence of intellectual deficits in MPTP-induced PD argues in favor of a specific cognitive change. The dementia cannot be clinically distinguished from AD, although late in PD, patients may exhibit frontal lobe deficits.

### Progressive Supranuclear Palsy

Progressive supranuclear palsy (PSP) is frequently characterized by dementia with prominent frontal lobe deficits, including emotional lability, frontal release signs (grasp, snout), and motor impersistence. The symptoms that bring patients to medical attention relate to their movement disorder, including supranuclear ophthalmoplegia (see Chapter 3), rigidity, and gait difficulty.

Lesions in the substantia nigra and globus pallidus are probably responsible for the rigidity and ataxia. Lesions in the pretectal nuclei, periaqueductal grey, and superior colliculi are responsible for the ocular motor abnormalities. Cerebral degeneration with pathological features that differ somewhat from those seen with AD is associated with intellectual decline.

### Huntington's Disease

Patients with Huntington's disease (HD) develop typical subcortical dementia, which is probably due to both striatal and frontal lobe neuronal loss. Diagnosis requires the presence of typical HD features, including chorea involving both sides; this finding makes a focal structural lesion unlikely. Family history is positive unless history or parentage is in dispute; the penetrance is high and the rate of new mutations is low. Occasional patients present with rigidity without chorea; this finding is especially common in patients with juvenile-onset HD.

## VISUAL FIELD ABNORMALITIES

### Anatomy

Visual input is transduced into action potentials in the eye. The information is then conducted via the optic nerves to the optic chiasm, where crossing of the hemifields occurs. The optic tracts carry information from the contralateral hemifields of both eyes to the lateral geniculate, where elementary visual processing is performed. Outflow from the lateral geniculate projects to the occipital cortex via the optic radiations. The optic radiations can be divided into two sections, one carrying information from the superior quadrant (inferior aspect of the retina) and one from the inferior quadrant (superior aspect of the retina). The portion of the optic radiation corresponding to the superior quadrant travels through the white matter of the temporal lobe in an arc (Meyer's loop). The effect of lesions at each level of the visual system is reported in Table 1.8 and shown in Figure 1.5.

**Cortical Visual Areas**

With clear-cut visual field abnormalities, localization is fairly straightforward, but with visual–perceptive and visual–associative problems the localization is less precise. The following are the major types of visual defects:

- Field defects
- Blindness
- Alexia
- Hallucinations

**Table 1.8    Visual Field Defects**

| Field Defect | Location | Typical Cause |
|---|---|---|
| Right hemianopia | Left optic tract, optic radiation, or occipital lobe | Compressive lesion, left MCA stroke, left PCA stroke |
| Macular-sparing right hemianopia | Occipital lobe; pole supplied by MCA spared | Left PCA stroke, macular region supplied by MCA |
| Right superior quadrant defect | Left temporal lobe and Meyer's loop | Left MCA stroke involving inferior division |
| Bitemporal hemianopia | Chiasmal lesion | Pituitary tumor |
| Binasal hemianopia | Chiasmal or perichiasmal lesion | Parasellar lesion, especially tumor |
| Incongruous field defect (junctional scotoma) | Chiasmal or perichiasmal lesion | Pituitary or parasellar lesion, especially tumor |

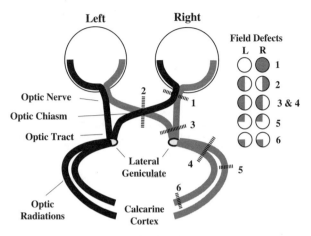

**Fig. 1.5** Pathways from the eye to brain are shown, along with effects of lesions on each.

Field defects are areas of loss of visual perception. The patient is often unaware of the deficit, so this sign is often found in the absence of symptoms, except perhaps a vague complaint of "blurry vision."

Cortical blindness is characterized by unawareness of the defect, along with confabulation. A common cause is occlusion of the basilar artery with secondary posterior cerebral artery occlusion (top-of-the-basilar syndrome). Patients present with cortical blindness—or with a lesser visual defect if they have incomplete lesions—plus a defect in short-term memory. The denial of blindness, also know as Anton's syndrome, is also seen in many patients with occipital infarction. Somnolence may be present, and pupillary and ocular motor defects may occur from midbrain ischemia.

Alexia is the inability to read due to interference with the input from the visual cortex to the auditory association areas in the left hemisphere. To produce alexia, a lesion must affect projections from both occipital lobes; that is, there may be simultaneous lesions of the ipsilateral calcarine cortex and the splenium of the corpus callosum (which is the route by which information gets to the left hemisphere from the right occipital region), or there may be a single lesion in the white matter deep to the parieto-occipital region, adjacent to the occipital horn of the lateral ventricle. The latter type of lesion can affect the projections of both occipital areas to the temporoparietal regions. Alexia in this sense refers to relatively purely alexia, without agraphia; a patient with severe language disorders due to an extensive left hemisphere lesion will have alexia, but it will be secondary to the language deficit rather than primary.

Hallucinations are common in patients with cortical lesions. Occipital lesions produce hallucinations composed of primitive visual patterns, such as colors and simple shapes. Temporal lobe lesions may produce hallucinations of more definite images, such as animals or people.

## VISUOSPATIAL DYSFUNCTION

The following are the major forms of visuospatial dysfunction:

- Constructional apraxia
- Neglect
- Apraxia

Constructional apraxia, discussed previously, is the inability to draw or copy a figure with spatial significance. To copy figures, the individual does not copy each line verbatim, but rather synthesizes a concept in the brain of what the figure should look like. If the centers concerning visuospatial orientation are not intact, the figures will be drawn incorrectly, frequently lacking the three-dimensional quality. The patient is often aware of the error but cannot fix it. Lesions producing constructional apraxia are classically in the right hemisphere, although left hemisphere and diffuse cerebral lesions can also result in constructional difficulties. The parietal cortex is predominantly involved in patients with constructional difficulties.

Neglect is the misperception of space; the patient with neglect ignores half of the universe, as if it did not exist. Neglect often includes misperception of the body, so that the patient does not recognize one side as being self or denies the existence of that half altogether. Patients with right parietal lesions often deny their left hemiparesis or that limbs held in front of them are their own. If one side of the body is not completely ignored, body image may be distorted in some other way. Neglect is usually due to a right hemisphere lesion, with prominence in the parietal region. Occasional patients with left hemisphere lesions will have some right-sided neglect.

As already discussed, apraxia also includes disorders of visuospatial function.

# 2

# Basal Ganglia and Thalamus

## BASAL GANGLIA

### Anatomy

The basal ganglia are composed of the following deep nuclei, which have complex interrelationships:

- Globus pallidus
- Putamen
- Caudate nucleus
- Subthalamic nucleus
- Claustrum
- Substantia nigra

The striatum consists of the putamen and caudate nucleus. The lentiform nucleus consists of the globus pallidus and putamen; it is called "lentiform" because its geometry is similar to that of an optical lens.

The basal ganglia are mainly involved in control of movement, especially the automatic components of locomotion and posture. While fine movements probably are initiated in the cortex, the basal ganglia are involved in feedback control of movements.

Figure 2.1 shows some important components of the basal ganglia and their interrelationship with other cerebral structures. Figure 2.2 shows basic connections between the basal ganglia and other brain regions; only the clinically most important connections are shown.

Major inputs to the basal ganglia are from the cerebral cortex, thalamus, and brain stem. Major outputs from the brain stem are from the globus pallidus to the ventral anterior (VA) and ventrolat-

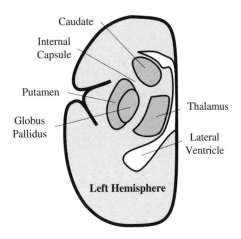

**Fig. 2.1** Axial section of the left cerebral hemisphere shows the relationships of parts of the basal ganglia to other structures.

eral (VL) nuclei of the thalamus; the thalamus projects back to the cerebral cortex as well.

Interconnections between the nuclei in the basal ganglia are plentiful; the following are some of the most important:

- From the substantia nigra to the striatum
- Between the substantia nigra and globus pallidus in both directions
- From the striatum to the globus pallidus
- Between the subthalamus and globus pallidus in both directions

With these afferent, efferent, and associative connections, some important circuits involve the following:

Cerebral cortex → striatum → thalamus → cerebral cortex
Striatum → globus pallidus → substantia nigra → striatum
Globus pallidus → subthalamic nucleus and back

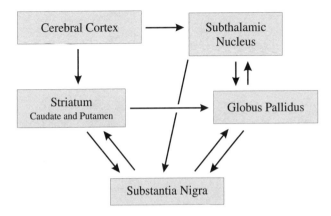

**Fig. 2.2** Some of the most important connections between elements of the basal ganglia and other brain centers are shown.

Circuits in the basal ganglia are probably involved in execution of patterned movements and error checking. The motor system can be thought of as a hierarchical network of controls. At the top is the cortex, which determines the focus and intent of the movement; at this level, the movement may be a concept rather than action of individual muscles and muscle groups. Output from the cortex projects to the basal ganglia, brain stem, and spinal cord. The purpose of the brain stem and spinal cord is to decode the intent to move into individual muscle movements, activating specific motoneurons and receiving feedback on the success of the intended movements.

The cerebellum receives input on movement and provides information used to correct movement. The basal ganglia also receive input regarding success of movement; however, unlike brain stem and cerebellar and spinal centers, the basal ganglia project their output predominantly to the cortex, which, in turn, modifies its output in accordance with the information received.

## Lesions

Lesions of the basal ganglia typically produce movement disorders, with the predominant results being abnormalities of tone and involuntary movement. For clinical purposes, the important classification is into the following two categories:

- Akinetic rigid syndromes
- Involuntary spontaneous movements

"Akinetic" refers to the lack of movement and "rigid" refers to muscle stiffness. Important entities in this category are Parkinson's disease, drug-induced parkinsonism, progressive supranuclear palsy, and striatonigral degeneration (Table 2.1). The differential diagnosis includes paratonia, which is increased muscle tone due to cerebral cortical damage, particularly in the frontal region. Involuntary spontaneous movements include essential tremor, Parkinson's tremor, dystonia, dyskinesias, chorea, athetosis, and hemiballismus.

It is impossible to classify each disease purely into one category. For example, Parkinson's disease is mainly an akinetic rigid syndrome, but tremor is an important feature. Huntington's disease presents with chorea in adults, but it may present with rigidity with juvenile onset.

### *Akinetic Rigid Syndromes*

*Parkinson's Disease*

Parkinson's disease (PD) is characterized by rigidity, bradykinesia, and tremor; however, not all of these may be present, especially early in the course. Gait is stooped with decreased arm swing. Steps are small and slow when the patient begins to walk but accelerate with distance (festination), predisposing the patient to falling down. Facial expression is reduced. Writing becomes smaller. The tremor is most prominent at rest, most prominent in the arms, and averages 4 to 5 hertz. Rigidity and tremor are often asymmetric early in the course. Late in the course, abnormalities in postural reflexes make ambulation hazardous.

Approximately 30 percent of people with PD have dementia; in some it may be the coexistence of Alzheimer's disease with PD, but

**Table 2.1   Akinetic Rigid Syndromes**

| Disorder | Features |
|---|---|
| Parkinson's disease | Bradykinesia, rigidity, resting tremor, postural disturbance |
| Drug-induced parkinsonism | Bradykinesia, rigidity, and postural instability, usually with less tremor than in Parkinson's disease |
| Striato-nigral degeneration | Bradykinesia and rigidity with less tremor than in Parkinson's disease; diagnosis is suggested by poor response to dopaminergic agents |
| Progressive supranuclear palsy | Rigidity, gait difficulty, and supranuclear ocular motor abnormalities, especially of vertical gaze |
| Shy-Drager syndrome | Parkinsonism, orthostatic hypotension, and other autonomic signs; other neurologic deficits common, including corticospinal tract signs, lower motoneuron degeneration, and/or cerebellar signs |
| Olivopontocerebellar atrophy (some clinicians classify this as a cerebellar degeneration) | Cerebellar signs associated with parkinsonism, dementia, peripheral neuropathy |
| Multiple system atrophy (term not used by some clinicians) | Orthostatic hypotension and other signs of autonomic failure, with parkinsonism, corticospinal tract signs, and cerebellar signs |

there appears to be a defined PD–dementia complex different from the hereditary PD–dementia complex found in Guam. (See below and Chapter 1.)

Tremor of PD is often confused with essential tremor. Distinguishing features are discussed in the section on essential tremor, below.

Drug-induced parkinsonism differs from classic PD because of its lesser degree of tremor, but clinical differentiation may be impossible. A history of drug use, especially neuroleptics, is present in patients with drug-induced parkinsonism. Parkinsonism can develop from MPTP exposure in drug abusers.

The differential diagnosis of idiopathic PD includes all of the other akinetic rigid syndromes discussed in this section, plus frontal lobe damage, which can result in a shuffling gait and lack of initiative; these symptoms may be mistaken for parkinsonism. All patients with parkinsonism must be asked specifically about neuroleptic exposure. Examination should detail the severity and distribution of the tremor, rigidity, bradykinesia, and gait and postural instability, not only to aid with diagnosis, but also for the purpose of future comparisons during treatment.

*Diffuse Lewy Body Disease*
Some patients with parkinsonian features will present with dementia early in the course. Aphasia and apraxia are common. Pathologically, Lewy bodies are distributed diffusely through the cortex rather than having a restricted distribution.

*Striatonigral Degeneration*
Striatonigral degeneration is characterized by rigidity and bradykinesia with less tremor than seen in idiopathic PD. The diagnosis is often suspected when the patient does not respond to dopaminergic agents. No clinical features can clearly distinguish striatonigral degeneration from more typical PD, and diagnosis is only confirmed at autopsy.

*Progressive Supranuclear Palsy*
Progressive supranuclear palsy (PSP) is characterized by rigidity, gait difficulty with a tendency to fall, and prominent ocular motor abnormalities. The ocular motor abnormalities are supranuclear in that the patient has impaired voluntarily gaze, but doll's-head maneuvers reveal preserved eye movement with passive turning of the head, at least early in the course. Vertical gaze is most prominently affected, with involvement of horizontal gaze late in the course. The supranuclear deficit extends not only to ocular movement, but also other brain stem functions. Patients will have dysarthria and dysphagia. Eventually, degeneration of the brain stem results in

deficits that cannot be overcome by reflexive maneuvers. Dementia is common, though usually mild.

The degeneration is not confined to the deep nuclei. Areas affected include substantia nigra, globus pallidus, subthalamic nuclei, periaqueductal gray, superior colliculus, and pretectal nuclei. Neuroanatomical localization is less important than recognition of the clinical syndrome for diagnosis.

### *Tremor*

The most common tremors are essential tremor, Parkinson's tremor, and enhanced physiologic tremor (Table 2.2). Essential tremor is most prominent with action; Parkinson's tremor is most prominent at rest; enhanced physiologic tremor is noted by patients during episodes of anxiety. Anxiety may exacerbate essential tremor, as well.

An action tremor can develop with cerebellar damage; it us accompanied by a characteristic incoordination of movement. Cerebellar damage is seldom confused with PD or essential tremor.

#### *Essential Tremor*

Essential tremor (ET) is most prominent with action and less apparent at rest. Stress exacerbates the tremor, leading some patients

**Table 2.2 Tremor**

| Disorder | Diagnosis |
| --- | --- |
| Parkinson's tremor | Tremor of 4–5 Hz most prominent at rest and less so with action; associated with other signs of parkinsonism |
| Essential tremor | Tremor of 5–8 Hz with action; little or no tremor at rest; no associated neurologic findings |
| Enhanced physiological tremor | High-frequency tremor with posture and movement, exacerbated by fatigue, anxiety, and many medications; no associated neurologic findings |
| Cerebellar tremor | Tremor of 3 Hz, mainly in a horizontal plane and most prominent with fine repetitive action of the extremities; associated with other signs of cerebellar ataxia |

and physicians to call it "nervous tremor." Ethanol suppresses the tremor, and some patients become alcoholics as a result. The tremor is most prominent in the hands, although the head is frequently affected, producing titubation. Voice tremor may occur.

Misdiagnosis of ET as parkinsonism by nonneurologists is among the most common errors in clinical practice. The two are differentiated by the effect of action on the tremor: ET is most prominent with movement or posture of the arms, while Parkinson's tremor is most prominent at rest. The frequency of ET is 5 to 8 hertz, faster than the 4 to 5 hertz of PD. Also, other findings of parkinsonism, such as rigidity, bradykinesia, and loss of postural reflexes, are not found.

*Parkinson's Tremor*
Tremor associated with Parkinson's disease is most prominent at rest and has a frequency of 4 to 5 hertz. The tremor is damped by action, but it is often still present. Associated neurologic findings of parkinsonism include bradykinesia, rigidity, positive glabellar reflexes, and impaired postural reflexes.

*Enhanced Physiologic Tremor*
Enhanced physiologic tremor is a high-frequency tremor that is most prominent with posture and action. It is exacerbated by anxiety, fatigue, and many drugs. Some of the most important provocative drugs and toxins are valproic acid, lithium, beta-agonists, theophylline, heavy metals, caffeine, and neuroleptics. Tremor associated with alcohol withdrawal is also enhanced physiological tremor.

## Dystonia and Dyskinesia
Dystonia is an abnormality of tone. Dyskinesia is a fragmentation of spontaneous movements. Athetosis, chorea, ballism, and tremor are abnormal spontaneous movements that, strictly speaking, fit under the heading of "dyskinesia." Athetosis is a slow writhing movement, most prominent distally. Chorea is a rapid jerky movement, mainly of distal muscles, that patients frequently blend into voli-

tional activity. Ballism is violent flinging movements; the unilateral version is hemiballismus.

Tremor is discussed separately, above, because it is usually clinically isolated from the other dyskinesias. Important causes of chorea and athetosis are presented in Table 2.3.

The possible causes of dystonia are many, but the most important can be broken down into the following classes:

- Structural
- Degenerative
- Metabolic
- Drug-induced
- Idiopathic

Structural causes include infarction, hemorrhage, tumor, abscess, vascular malformation, postsurgical complications, and trauma. Degenerative causes include Huntington's disease, PD, progressive supranuclear palsy, and olivopontocerebellar atrophy. Dopa-responsive dystonia probably falls into this category.

Metabolic causes include Wilson's disease, some amino acid defects, metachromatic leukodystrophy, Hallervorden–Spatz disease, Leigh disease, ataxia telangiectasia, Niemann–Pick disease, and Lesch–Nyhan syndrome. Drug-induced dystonia is most often due to neuroleptics, but it can also be due to dopamine agonists used for treatment of parkinsonism.

Idiopathic dystonia includes several syndromes that may ultimately be found to belong in the degenerative or metabolic categories:

- Dystonia musculorum deformans
- Dopa-responsive dystonia
- Paroxysmal dystonia
- Focal dystonias, including writer's cramp, cranial dystonia, and torticollis

*Dystonia Musculorum Deformans*
Dystonia musculorum deformans is a generalized dystonia, but it often begins in one extremity, such as turning of the foot. Over

**Table 2.3    Chorea and Athetosis**

| Disorder | Features |
| --- | --- |
| Basal ganglia lesion, including infarction or mass lesion | Unilateral chorea, usually associated with weakness and incoordination |
| Carbon monoxide poisoning | Basal ganglia damage, which produces bilateral chorea; often associated with signs of cerebral demyelination and history of exposure |
| Chorea gravidarum | Chorea during pregnancy, rarely associated with rheumatic fever, more frequently with SLE; related to chorea with oral contraceptives |
| Drug-induced chorea | History of use of oral contraceptives, phenytoin, dopamine agonists, neuroleptics, and/or anti-cholinergics; patients with previous Sydenham's chorea especially susceptible |
| Calcification of the basal ganglia | Usually asymptomatic, but possible chorea, parkinsonism, dystonia; diagnosis by CT |
| Hallervorden–Spatz disease | Progressive choreoathetosis or parkinsonism in childhood, often with dystonia; abnormalities on MRI in the globus pallidus |
| Huntington's disease | Autosomal dominant chorea beginning in the hands, exacerbated by movement and walking and associated with ocular motor abnormalities, psychiatric disorder; family history and imaging aid diagnosis |
| Paroxysmal choreoathetosis | Episodic onset of chorea and/or dystonia; no symptoms between episodes |
| SLE | Unilateral or bilateral chorea, often with a history of chorea during pregnancy or history of fetal loss; possible features of collagen vascular disease; positive ANA |
| Sydenham's chorea | Unilateral or bilateral chorea with onset in youth; history of recent streptococcal infection |
| Wilson's disease | Chorea uncommon; psychiatric abnormalities, dystonia, rigidity, tremor, and hepatic findings more typical |

SLE = systemic lupus erythematosus; CT = computerized tomography; MRI = magnetic resonance imaging; ANA = antinuclear antibody.

time, other muscles are affected; eventually, most body muscles are involved. Dystonia affecting proximal muscles, including those of the trunk, interferes with gait, producing body postures during walking that can resemble those seen in adults with cerebral palsy. The gait may be so bizarre that the cause is mistakenly believed to be psychiatric. Progression is expected.

Onset is typically in childhood; the problem is often thought to be a focal dystonia until more generalized signs develop. Focal dystonias are much less likely to progress to generalized dystonia in adults.

### Dopa-Responsive Dystonia

Dopa-responsive dystonia begins in childhood with progressive dystonia first affecting the legs. There is a 2:1 female predominance. Average age of onset is 6 years. The dystonia is worse late in the day and better after sleep.

Identification of patients with dopa-responsive dystonias is important because they respond to low doses of L-dopa. This disorder may be present in up to 10 percent of children who present with idiopathic dystonia; therefore, it is reasonable to try L-dopa in all such patients.

### Focal Dystonias

Spasmodic torticollis is the most common focal dystonia. Patients present with involuntary head turning or tilting. Initially, the movements are intermittent, but they subsequently become persistent. Patients often learn that a light touch on the face can cause the head to turn back to the primary position. Pain from sustained muscle contraction is common. The exact lesion responsible for torticollis is not known, but basal ganglion dysfunction has been implicated.

Blepharospasm is characterized by forced eye closure with depression of the eye brows. It begins with frequent blinking and is only recognized by patients when sustained eyelid closure impairs vision.

Oromandibular dystonia can take a variety of forms, including forced tongue protrusion and jaw opening or closing, often with dysarthria and dysphagia. Spasmodic dysphonia is due to involuntary contraction of laryngeal muscles. Meige syndrome is blepharospasm with oromandibular dystonia.

Writer's cramp is one of the occupational focal dystonias. It is characterized by muscular contraction of intrinsic muscles of the hand, and it is exacerbated by writing and other fine movements.

*Huntington's Disease*

Huntington's disease (HD) is characterized by choreiform movements, most prominent in the hands, that are exacerbated by movement, including walking. The chorea becomes generalized later in the course of the disease. Associated neurologic findings include ocular motor dysfunctions such as saccadic pursuit, gaze impersistence, and convergence paresis. Tongue protrusion is common. Psychiatric abnormalities include personality change, psychosis, and ultimately dementia.

Diagnosis is supported by positive family history, brain scans showing atrophy of the caudate nucleus, and genetic testing. Counseling is performed prior to genetic testing to ensure that the patient understands the implications of the diagnosis. I do not encourage my patients to undergo genetic testing.

Degeneration is widespread in HD, with cortical and subcortical atrophy; therefore, HD cannot be thought of as having a focal anatomic localization. The gene is localized to chromosome 4. HD is inherited as autosomal dominant with absolute penetrance; the frequency of new mutations is much lower than the frequency of uncertain parentage. HD shows anticipation—that is, clinical manifestations appear earlier in successive generations. Patients with HD at a young age commonly present with rigidity rather than chorea.

*Sydenham's Chorea*

Sydenham's chorea presents with typical choreiform movements, which last for a week or weeks then abate. Occasional patients will have recurrent bouts of chorea. Most patients are children between 5 and 15 years of age. Most but not all patients will have a prior history of rheumatic fever. This disorder has become rare with the increasing use of antibiotics effective against group A streptococcal infections.

*Wilson's Disease*
Wilson's disease is an defect in copper metabolism with autosomal recessive inheritance. Copper accumulates in the liver, brain, cornea, and other organs, and the resultant liver disease produces nausea, vomiting, anorexia, malaise, and weight loss. Neurologic involvement causes personality change, affective disturbance, dystonia, tremor, rigidity, dysarthria, and gait difficulties.

Wilson's disease should be considered in young individuals with a movement disorder, unexplained liver disease, and personality change; obviously, not all depressed individuals should be screened for Wilson's disease. Diagnosis is supported by a Kayser–Fleischer ring in the cornea on slit-lamp examination. Serum ceruloplasmin concentration is usually low, but occasional patients may have levels in the normal range. Liver biopsy can confirm copper accumulation but is usually not necessary. Brain imaging shows degeneration of the basal ganglia plus cortical atrophy with compensatory ventricular dilatation.

*Athetoid Cerebral Palsy*
Many patients with cerebral palsy present with prominent mental retardation and spasticity. In contrast, patients with athetoid cerebral palsy present with choreoathetosis, dystonia, and myoclonus and with less intellectual dysfunction than seen in patients with prominent cortical involvement.

*Kernicterus*
Kernicterus is characterized by choreoathetosis with dystonia, often accompanied by mental retardation, oculomotor abnormalities, and spasticity. Kernicterus closely resembles athetoid cerebral palsy.

## Hallervorden–Spatz Disease

Hallervorden–Spatz disease presents in childhood with progressive choreoathetosis or parkinsonism. Dystonia is common early in the course. Adult-onset Hallervorden–Spatz disease often presents as parkinsonism. Iron is deposited in the globus pallidus, the pars reticularis of the substantia nigra, and the red nucleus.

Diagnosis is considered in children with progressive choreoathetosis, parkinsonism, or dystonia. Magnetic resonance imaging shows abnormal areas of low signal, most prominently in the globus pallidus, on T2-weighted images. Computerized tomography is usually not helpful.

## Paroxysmal Choreoathetosis

Paroxysmal choreoathetosis begins in childhood; it is characterized by episodic chorea or dystonia that has a defined beginning and end. The disorder can be divided into two subsets, depending on whether the paroxysms are kinesigenic (that is, triggered by movement): paroxysmal kinesigenic choreoathetosis and paroxysmal nonkinesigenic choreoathetosis. Both often show autosomal recessive inheritance and mostly affect males.

Paroxysmal kinesigenic choreoathetosis starts in childhood and is characterized by movement-induced paroxysms that usually last five minutes or less. Paroxysmal nonkinesigenic choreoathetosis starts in infancy and is not triggered by movement. Paroxysms can last for hours.

No clear-cut pathologic localization has been identified with these disorders. Identification of the paroxysmal dyskinesias is important because of their occasional response to benzodiazepines and anticonvulsants.

## Tardive Dyskinesia

Tardive dyskinesia (TD) is characterized by repetitive orolingual movements including lip smacking, tongue protrusion, and chewing movements. Limb muscles may be involved, giving the appearance of chorea.

TD develops after prolonged neuroleptic exposure. Unlike other neuroleptic-induced syndromes, such as parkinsonism and malignant neuroleptic syndrome, TD may persist following discontinuation of the neuroleptic; it may actually appear to worsen shortly after discontinuation of the drug.

The location of the lesion producing TD is not completely known. One hypothesis suggests that there is supersensitivity of the dopamine receptors in the striatum.

*Hemifacial Spasm*
Hemifacial spasm is a disorder of the facial nerve that can be mistaken for paroxysmal dyskinesia. It is discussed in Chapter 3.

*Hemiballismus*
Damage to the subthalamic nucleus is thought to be the cause of hemiballismus, which is characterized by violent movements of the contralateral limbs, mainly through the proximal muscles. The limbs have a flinging appearance. Smaller distal movements are common as well, creating a continuum between ballism and chorea. The distal movements have more of the appearance of chorea.

The most common cause of hemiballismus is infarction. Other important causes include tumor, hemorrhage, and demyelination plaque from multiple sclerosis.

## THALAMUS

### Anatomy

The thalamus has many functions, although its basic task is processing afferent information. The ventroposterior (VP) nuclear complex is the main somesthetic receiving area; it consists of the ventroposterolateral (VPL) and ventroposteromedial (VPM) nuclei. Ascending information from the head and face projects to the VPM nuclei, while input from the rest of the body projects to VPL nuclei. The VP complex projects mainly to the primary somatosensory region of the cortex on the postcentral gyrus (areas 1, 2, and 3).

The exception is taste, which ascends to VPM nuclei and projects to the ventral aspect of the precentral gyrus, adjacent to the insula.

More specifically, the posterior nuclear group receives nociceptive input from the spinothalamic tracts and projects to the secondary somesthetic region on the inner aspect of the postcentral cortex, adjacent to the insula.

The VA nucleus receives input from the substantia nigra and globus pallidus as well as from other thalamic nuclei, brain stem reticular formation, and cerebral cortex. Projections are to the premotor area of the frontal lobe (area 6) and the supplementary motor area on the superior frontal gyrus (also area 6). The VA nucleus is probably involved in processing the information that causes alerting. Damage to this area results in decreased alertness and inattention, which can resemble frontal lobe deficits.

The VL nucleus receives input from the cerebellum, substantia nigra, and globus pallidus. In addition, it receives lesser input from the cerebral cortex, reticular formation, and other thalamic nuclei. The VL nucleus has projections to and from the primary motor cortex on the precentral gyrus (area 4). It is involved in control over movement, and it is an integral part of two control loops:

Cerebellar loop: cerebral cortex → pons → cerebellum → red nucleus → thalamus → cerebral cortex

Basal ganglia loop: cerebral cortex → basal ganglia → thalamus → cerebral cortex

Damage to the cerebellar loop results in predominantly cerebellar ataxia. Damage to the basal ganglia loop results in extrapyramidal findings, including parkinsonism, dystonia, and dyskinesias.

The medial geniculate body receives auditory input from the brain stem, especially the inferior colliculus. Projections are to the auditory cortex on the superior temporal gyrus (area 41).

The lateral geniculate body receives visual input via the optic tracts. Since the lateral geniculate is central to the optic chiasm, the lateral geniculate conveys information from the contralateral visual hemifield. There are six layers, with each layer relaying information from only one eye; the ipsilateral eye fibers project to layers 2, 3, and 5, and the contralateral eye fibers project to layers 1, 4, and 6. Projections are via the optic radiations to the primary visual cortex (area 17) on the medial aspect of the occipital lobe.

## Lesions

Important syndromes due predominantly to thalamic dysfunction are summarized in Table 2.4. Other disorders implicate the thalamus, but the clinical findings are not restricted to the thalamus.

### *Thalamic Infarction*

The thalamus is supplied mainly by branches of the posterior cerebral artery with some supply from posterior communicating arteries. The vessels enter the substance of the thalamus in a manner similar to that of the lenticulostriate vessels. In some individuals, the vessels to both sides arise from one posterior cerebral artery; in this circumstance, unilateral vascular lesion can result in bilateral thalamic infarction.

Infarction of the thalamus may produce varied symptoms depending on the exact regions affected. Common symptoms include

**Table 2.4   Thalamic Syndromes**

| Syndrome | Features |
|---|---|
| Thalamic infarction | Contralateral sensory loss, sometimes with motor, speech, and behavioral disorders; left hemisphere lesions produce more prominent language disturbance including aphasia; right hemisphere lesions can produce neglect |
| Thalamic pain | Contralateral pain exacerbated by stimulation; sensory detection thresholds are increased |

contralateral hemisensory loss, thalamic pain syndrome (see below), and motor deficit (see below).

Since the thalamus is supplied by the posterior circulation, associated findings often include midbrain damage from infarction in a basilar distribution and/or hemianopia due to posterior cerebral artery occlusion. Infarction in the anterior circulation (that is, the branches of the internal carotid, including the middle cerebral artery) do not produce thalamic damage.

### Thalamic Sensory Disorders

The sensory deficit from thalamic infarction can affect the entire contralateral body, including face, arm, leg, and trunk. Other findings include neglect, which may resemble that seen with parietal lobe damage of the right hemisphere damage.

#### Thalamic Pain Syndrome

Thalamic pain syndrome is characterized by severe pain contralateral to a lesion in the thalamus. The pain is present at rest but exacerbated by sensory stimulation. Sensory detection thresholds are elevated. Infarction is the most common cause of thalamic pain. Involvement of the posterior ventrobasal region is thought to be necessary for generation of thalamic pain.

### Mental Status Changes

In occasional patients with dementia and decreased levels of consciousness, the main finding on laboratory studies is bilateral degeneration of the thalamus. There are often associated eye findings, including pupillary abnormalities. Patients with top-of-the-basilar syndrome present with deficits in short-term memory associated with cortical blindness.

### Language Disorders

Language disturbance can develop after dominant hemisphere thalamic infarction. Patients develop a transcortical aphasia with impaired naming, word searching, and word substitution but preserved repetition. The transcortical feature of this language disturbance is helpful in differentiating thalamic from cortical lesions. The aphasia is usually transient.

## *Motor Disorders*

Patients with thalamic lesions are not paralyzed, but they often have difficulty moving; this difficulty probably reflects connection of the thalamus with the basal ganglia. This finding is most common with lesions that involve the ventrothalamic and subthalamic regions. Formal testing reveals essentially normal strength of muscles when they are tested individually, but there is decreased tone and a tendency to not use the muscles voluntarily (a form of neglect). This condition is likely due to a deficit in the sensory feedback responsible for maintaining normal movement.

# 3

# Cranial Nerves, Brain Stem, and Cerebellum

It is impossible to completely separate the anatomy of the cranial nerves, brain stem, and cerebellum, since all are centered in the posterior fossa and have strong functional and structural interconnections. However, to aid in comprehension, this chapter discusses cranial nerves, brain stem, and cerebellar anatomy and lesions individually, followed by coverage of syndromes that commonly affect more than one division.

## CRANIAL NERVES

Cranial nerves are discussed individually except for the oculomotor, trochlear, and abducens, which together control ocular movement. Lesions affecting one cranial nerve solely or predominantly are discussed under the respective nerve; brain stem lesions producing cranial nerve dysfunction in addition to other neurologic dysfunctions are discussed at the end of the chapter. Table 3.1 summarizes cranial nerve function. Figure 3.1 shows external brain stem anatomy and exit sites of the cranial nerves.

### Olfactory Nerve

#### Anatomy

The sensory receptors of the olfactory nerve are located at the superior aspect of the nasal cavity. Multiple small fiber bundles enter the cranial vault through the cribriform plate and then enter the olfactory bulb where they synapse on the second-order neurons. The axons travel posteriorly through the olfactory tract beneath the frontal lobes. In the region of the optic chiasm, the olfactory

**Table 3.1    Cranial Nerves**

| Number | Name | Motor Function | Sensory Function |
|--------|------|----------------|------------------|
| I | Olfactory | | Smell |
| II | Optic | | Vision |
| III | Oculomotor | Superior, inferior, and medial recti, inferior oblique; pupil and ciliary muscles | |
| IV | Trochlear | Superior oblique | |
| V | Trigeminal | Mastication of muscles | Controls face, forehead, external ear, mucosa, cornea, sinuses |
| VI | Abducens | Lateral rectus | |
| VII | Facial | Muscles of face and scalp; stapedius | Innervates soft palate; controls taste of anterior two thirds of tongue |
| VIII | Vestibulo-cochlear | | Innervates hearing; Controls position in space; acceleration |
| IX | Glosso-pharyngeal | Pharyngeal muscles; stylopharyngeus muscle | Innervates pharynx; controls taste to posterior two thirds of tongue |
| X | Vagus | Pharynx, larynx; thoracic and abdominal viscera | Controls pharynx, larynx, external auditory canal, thoracic and abdominal viscera |
| XI | Accessory | Sternocleidomastoid, trapezius, some pharynx, upper larynx | |
| XII | Hypoglossal | Tongue, strap muscles of the neck | |

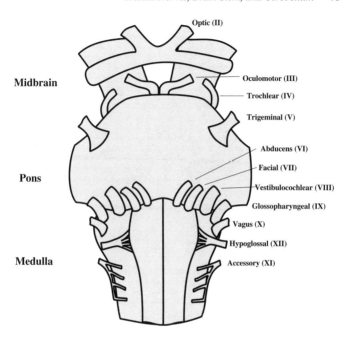

**Fig. 3.1** Ventral view of the brain stem and cranial nerves shows exit sites of the cranial nerves.

tracts divide into medial and lateral striae; some of the former decussate in the anterior commissure. The lateral stria project to temporal lobe.

### Lesions

Anosmia is produced by peripheral or central processes. Sinusitis can impair flow of air to the sensory regions. Head injury is a common cause of anosmia due to disruption of the small olfactory nerves that penetrate the cribriform plate.

Tumors of the olfactory grove compress the inferior frontal region, producing few neurologic signs. Patients may present with mood alteration. While patients rarely complain of olfactory abnormalities, examination reveals anosmia.

Other important causes of anosmia include increased intracranial pressure and some neurodegenerative diseases, including Parkinson's disease and Alzheimer's disease.

## Optic Nerve

### Anatomy

The retinal nerves that gather in the optic disk and exit the eye form the optic nerve. The nerve passes through the posterior aspect of the orbit and enters the skull through the optic canal. Nerve fibers serving the temporal field of each eye decussate at the optic chiasm. The optic tract exits the chiasm and projects to the lateral geniculate.

Optic nerve axons synapse in the lateral geniculate and project to the primary visual cortex. A small proportion of the fibers exit the lateral geniculate and project to the Edinger–Westphal nucleus in the midbrain to control pupil diameter.

### Lesions

Optic nerve lesions usually produce monocular visual loss, and subacute deficits may not be initially noticed by the patient. Formal testing may reveal reduced visual acuity that cannot be improved by correcting for refractive error. Color vision is often impaired. If a focal portion of the optic nerve is compressed or otherwise damaged, there may be a monocular abnormality in visual fields. Figure 1.5 (Chapter 1) shows changes in visual fields with lesions of the optic nerves, chiasm, and tracts. Important causes of optic neuropathy include the following:

- Optic neuritis
- Multiple sclerosis
- Tumors
- Trauma

Optic neuritis is characterized by inflammation and demyelination of the optic nerve. This finding is usually idiopathic, although approximately 30 percent of patients with optic neuritis subsequently develop multiple sclerosis (MS). Clinical features cannot clearly differentiate isolated optic neuritis from MS-associated optic neuritis.

For the diagnosis of MS, history or examination has to indicate evidence of other neurologic lesions that could be due to central demyelination. Magnetic resonance imaging (MRI) is helpful to rule out optic nerve compression and also to look for signs of white matter changes in the brain. See Chapter 1 for a discussion of the clinical criteria for multiple sclerosis.

The three most important tumors affecting the optic nerves and tracts are gliomas, meningiomas, and pituitary tumors. Optic nerve gliomas can occur as isolated entities or in association with neurofibromatosis. Patients present with progressive visual loss. The tumor location can be identified based on details of the visual fields. Proptosis (forward protrusion of the eye) suggests involvement of the nerve in the orbit, and pituitary tumors produce deformation of the optic chiasm, resulting in junctional scotomata.

Trauma commonly damages the eye or optic nerves, and detailed evaluation must be performed as soon as possible after the injury. Periorbital edema may make ocular examination impossible by 24 to 48 hours after the injury.

## Ocular Motor System

### *Anatomy*

The final pathway for eye movement begins in the brain stem with the midbrain and pontine nuclei; however, voluntary control of eye movement originates in the cerebral hemispheres. There are at least four basic types of eye movements:

- Pursuit movements
- Saccadic movements
- Vergence movements
- Corrective movements

Pursuit movements are synchronous movements of the eyes to follow a target that is moving relative to the head. Saccades are quick synchronous movements to direct attention at a new target. Vergence movements keep the target on the fovea of both eyes as it moves toward or away from the head. Corrective movements are small movements of the eyes produced by motion of the head in space; they depend on the vestibular system and feedback from smooth pursuit mechanisms.

### *Supranuclear Control of Eye Movement*

Pursuit mechanisms depend on input to the cortex about target location, direction of movement, and speed. Visual information from one hemifield is relayed to the contralateral visual cortex through subcortical pathways. While the pathways in humans are not completely known, visual information is believed to be relayed to the parieto-occipital region for processing into the target parameters mentioned above. This information is then sent to the frontal eye fields bilaterally.

Once the visual information is received and processed, the motor system acts to follow the target. Efferents from the frontal eye fields project to the pons and then to ocular motor nuclei. Efferents from visual processing areas also project to the pons, but output is relayed through the cerebellum, the medial vestibular nucleus, and then the ocular motor nuclei.

Pursuit eye movements are directed by the ipsilateral hemisphere—that is, pursuit to the left is directed by the left hemisphere. Pursuit therefore requires interaction between visual receiving areas in the occipital lobe, parietal and temporal association areas, and frontal eye fields. Commands to move are probably relayed via pontine nuclei to the ocular motor nuclei, bypassing the paramedian pontine reticular formation (PPRF).

Saccadic eye movements are fast conjugate movements that cause the eyes to acquire a new target. Activation of the left frontal eye fields in area 8 of the frontal lobe, posterior on the second frontal gyrus, produces a saccade to the right. This is mediated by projections from the frontal lobe to the PPRF.

Saccadic eye movements can also be induced by novel visual stimuli at the periphery of vision. The superior colliculus directly receives input from optic nerve fibers representing the contralateral visual field; this input triggers a saccade in the direction of the novel stimulus.

### Brain Stem Control of Eye Movement

PONTINE GAZE CENTERS

The PPRF is just lateral to the midline and adjacent to the sixth nerve nucleus. This region is responsible for lateral gaze. Descending input to the PPRF from the cerebral hemispheres directs gaze to the right or left. If right gaze is needed, the right PPRF is activated, and it in turn directs the ipsilateral sixth nerve (abducens) nucleus to activate the lateral rectus and abduct the right eye. Efferents from the PPRF cross to the contralateral side of the brain stem and ascend in the medial longitudinal fasciculus (MLF) to the midbrain where they direct the third nerve (oculomotor) nucleus to activate the medial rectus and adduct the left eye.

Lesion of the PPRF produces a lateral gaze palsy. Differentiation of a gaze palsy due to a cerebral lesion from one due to a brain stem lesion is aided by response to caloric stimulation—movement of the eyes in response to irrigation of the ear with cool water—and also by associated weakness. With a frontal lobe lesion, the eyes can be forced across the midline by calorics or doll's-head maneuvers; this finding points to a gaze preference rather than a gaze palsy. With a pontine lesion, the eyes cannot be forced across the midline, even with calorics, unless the lesion is incomplete. With both frontal and pontine lesions, weakness is contralateral; however, the gaze difficulty differs. With frontal lesions the eyes look toward the side of the lesion—that is, away from the paralyzed side; with a pontine lesion the eyes look away from the side of the lesion—that is, toward the side of the paralysis.

Lesion of the MLF produces internuclear ophthalmoplegia (INO). This is characterized by impaired adduction of the contralateral eye with gaze to one side. For example, with right gaze, the ipsilateral eye is abducted correctly, but the contralateral eye is not adducted. Because of the mismatch, the patient perceives diplopia with lateral gaze, when looking to the side opposite to the lesion, since the MLF is crossed. Nystagmus of the right (abducting) eye is common; the right eye returns toward the midline in an attempt to correct the diplopia, but then the PPRF forces the eye to abduct again. In practice, a strictly unilateral lesion of the MLF is unusual, because the two sides are both near the midline of the brain stem; bilateral INO presents with difficulty adducting either eye with lateral gaze. Occasionally, patients with INO are erroneously labeled as having sixth nerve palsies because of the diplopia with lateral gaze, but examination of the eye movements makes the distinction clear. The two most common causes of INO are MS and paramedian brain stem infarction.

MIDBRAIN CENTERS

The midbrain contains the nuclei of cranial nerve (CN) III and CN IV, which form a complex network responsible for their movement and also coordinates conjugate vertical movements, convergence, accommodation (change in lens shape for near focusing), and pupil diameter.

Input to the midbrain ascends and descends, as already discussed. Light reflex is caused by axons that project from the lateral geniculate to the Edinger–Westphal nucleus.

Vertical eye movements are mainly accomplished by activation of individual muscles innervated by CN III. Axons from the frontal lobes project to both CN III nuclei to evoke vertical movement. Convergence is initiated by a neuronal group in the midline of the midbrain; convergence causes activation of the medial recti, accommodation, and pupil constriction.

Pupil diameter is controlled by the combined action of constrictor and dilator muscles. Constrictor fibers are innervated by parasympathetic neurons that arise in the Edinger–Westphal nucleus and project to the eye via CN III. Dilator fibers are innervated by sympathetic neurons that arise in the hypothalamus and project through the brain stem and into the spinal cord, descending to the level of T1, where the sympathetic fibers exit and join the cervical sympathetic chain. In the neck, the axons leave the chain and ascend into the skull with the carotid artery. Axons innervating the eyelid join CN III for its final course. Axons innervating the pupil join the nasociliary nerve, a branch of CN V1, and then extend to the pupil via the long ciliary nerve.

Eyelid elevation is controlled jointly by sympathetic and CN III axons. The sympathetic axons have the course already described, and the course of the CN III axons is described below. Damage to either CN III or the sympathetic pathway can produce ptosis. Eyelid closure is accomplished by the orbicularis oculi, which are innervated by CN VII.

## Cranial Nerves Involved in Eye Movement
### OCULOMOTOR NERVE
The oculomotor nucleus lies medially in the midbrain, inferior to the aqueduct of Sylvius at the level of the superior colliculus. The nucleus is actually a complex; the most anterior portion is the Edinger–Westphal nucleus, which controls pupillary constriction by the sphincter of the iris and accommodation by the ciliary muscle. The rest of the oculomotor nerve complex controls the other third nerve muscles. The nuclei for the two sides are separate except for the Edinger–Westphal nucleus and the portion of the complex controlling the superior rectus; therefore, localized nuclear lesions affecting one side affect the other as well. The axons exit the midbrain between the cerebral peduncles and then pass through the cavernous sinus and the superior orbital fissure. At the fissure, the nerve divides into superior and inferior rami; the superior ramus innervates the superior rectus and lid levators, and the inferior ramus innervates the inferior rectus, inferior oblique, sphincter of the iris, and ciliary muscle.

### TROCHLEAR NERVE
The trochlear nucleus lies immediately caudal to the oculomotor nucleus at the level of the inferior colliculus. Axons cross the midline, then exit the midbrain on the dorsal surface near the inferior colliculus. The nerve turns around the brain stem to extend anteriorly, passing through the cavernous sinus and the superior or-

bital fissure. The superior oblique is the only muscle supplied by this nerve.

ABDUCENS NERVE

The abducens nucleus is located in the caudal pons. Motoneurons give rise to axons that course rostrally and medial to the facial nerve and nucleus, then turn to exit lateral to the corticospinal tract fibers at the pontomedullary junction. The axons then ascend ventral to the pons, travel on the lateral wall of the cavernous sinus, and enter the orbit through the superior orbital fissure. Interneurons in the abducens nucleus cross the midline and ascend to the midbrain in the MLF.

Abducens palsy presents with impaired lateral rectus function and decreased eye abduction. There is no ptosis, so the diplopia is obvious, in contrast to third nerve palsy. Important causes of CN VI palsy are increased intracranial pressure and small vessel disease (diabetes, hypertension); some cases are idiopathic. Sixth nerve palsy may be associated with mastoiditis, middle ear infection, and nasopharyngeal carcinomas with skull infiltration. Cavernous sinus thrombosis is associated with sixth nerve palsy with exophthalmos and periorbital pain. Sixth nerve lesion may occur with herpes zoster ophthalmicus; third nerve palsy can also occur. Lesions in the region of the superior orbital fissure may affect the sixth, third, and fourth nerves. Sixth nerve lesion may occur with minor infections, especially in children. Gradenigo's syndrome is from mastoid infection and is characterized by sixth, seventh, eighth, and occasionally fifth nerve lesions.

## Lesions

### Examination

Detailed eye movement examination is warranted in every patient with subjective diplopia or who has signs of an ocular motor defect on neurologic examination. The following should be done:

- Movements of each eye should be tested in all of the primary directions of gaze.
- Diplopia should be assessed with different directions of gaze.

- Pupillary responses to light and accommodation should be checked.
- The "swinging-flashlight test" should be done to test for an afferent pupil.

The eyes are tested together, although the examiner should concentrate on the specific responses of each eye. Nystagmus of one eye should prompt examination of the eyes individually. The examiner must use his knowledge of neuroanatomy during the examination to determine whether the defects are best explained by a defect in cranial nerves, brain stem, brain, or extraocular muscles.

The precision of eye movement may limit the ability of the examiner to detect subtle divergence of gaze; therefore, the patient should be asked about diplopia with directions of gaze. Pupillary response is elicited by shining a bright light into each eye of the patient, one eye at a time. The diameter of the each pupil before and during light exposure is noted. When the light is shone in one eye, both eyes should constrict equally.

The swinging-flashlight test examines pupillary responses from both eyes. The room must be dark enough that the eyes are not constricted, yet light enough that the diameter of the pupils can be determined. A bright light is shone first into one eye then quickly into the other. The normal response is constriction of both pupils when the light is initially shone into one eye. Quickly moving the light between the eyes should result in no alteration in diameter. If both pupils constrict more when light is shone into one eye than the other, the eye eliciting the lesser constriction is described as having an afferent defect, which points to an optic nerve or orbital lesion.

Optokinetic nystagmus (OKN) is elicited by the movement of a patterned background. The typical stimulus is passing scenery as a car drives through the country side. The eyes fix on an object of interest, and the image moves toward the rear of the vehicle. When fixation can no longer be maintained, gaze is redirected toward the front of the vehicle, and a new target is selected. The fast phase of the nystagmus is toward the front of the vehicle. In clinical practice, OKN is elicited by passing a striped tape in front of the eyes at a constant velocity. The nystagmus is analogous to the eye movements elicited by the vehicle movement. OKN is normally symmetric with movement of the tape in either direction. Lesion of one hemisphere in the parieto-occipital region produces an abnormal or absent OKN when the tape is moved toward the side of the lesion. An even more compelling stimulus is movement of a mirror held close in front of the patient. Compensatory movements are virtually impossible to suppress.

One of the most important uses of OKN is for diagnosis of psychogenic blindness. Patients who are blind will not develop OKN, whereas patients with psychogenic blindness often will.

*Differential Diagnosis of Ocular Motor Abnormalities*
Examination of the eyes is confounded if more than one cranial nerve is affected; while multiple cranial neuropathies must be considered, central lesions and neuromuscular lesions should be considered as well. The deficits associated with single lesions are listed in Table 3.2. Ocular motor defects and associated anatomic localizations are presented in Table 3.3.

*Cerebral Lesions*
The anatomy of cerebral control over eye movement is discussed earlier in this chapter. Massive lesions of one hemisphere are associated with a contralateral hemiparesis plus gaze preference to the side of the lesion—that is, the side opposite to the hemiparesis. With oculovestibular reflexes, the eyes can usually be brought across the midline. More restricted lesions of the hemisphere will result in smaller deficits, usually due to frontal lobe damage.

FRONTAL LOBE LESIONS
Frontal lobe lesions result in gaze preference to the side of the lesion. Since the hemisphere is also important for pursuit to the side of the lesion, pursuit is impaired as well. Surviving neurons may compensate for the gaze preference within hours if there are incomplete lesions; more typically, the gaze preference lasts days, then corrects.

Occasional patients are seen with eye deviation toward the side of the paralysis. These patients often have deep lesions involving the thalamus.

Frontal lobe irritative lesions affecting the frontal eye fields may cause paroxysms of gaze toward the side contralateral to the lesion. Seizures would be a typical example. Following the seizure, the gaze would likely be to the side ipsilateral to the lesion as a post-ictal phenomenon.

**Table 3.2  Focal Lesions Affecting the Ocular Motor System**

| Lesion | Findings |
| --- | --- |
| Left frontal lobe destructive lesion | Left gaze preference, often associated with right hemiparesis |
| Left frontal lobe irritative lesion (e.g., seizure) | Right gaze preference; sometimes associated with nystagmoid movements of eyes |
| Left parieto-occipital region lesion | Defective smooth pursuit in both horizontal directions of gaze in the contralateral hemifield |
| CN III palsy | Ptosis and impaired upward gaze and adduction; extrinsic compressive lesions affect pupil early; nerve ischemia often spares pupillary fibers |
| CN IV palsy | Impaired depression of the ipsilateral eye while in adduction; head tilt to side opposite lesion, due to slight external rotation of eye |
| CN VI palsy | Impaired abduction of ipsilateral eye |
| Medial longitudinal fasciculus | Internuclear ophthalmoplegia; impaired adduction of the ipsilateral eye with gaze to side opposite lesion; nystagmus of the contralateral (abducting) eye common |
| Pontine lesion (Millard–Gubler syndrome) | Ipsilateral CN VI palsy, facial palsy, and contralateral hemiparesis |
| Midbrain lesion (Parinaud's syndrome) | Impaired upgaze with dilated and nonreactive pupils |

CN = cranial nerve.

**Table 3.3  Localization of Ocular Motor Defects**

| Defect | Features | Localization and Type of Lesion |
| --- | --- | --- |
| Downbeat nystagmus | Vertical nystagmus with fast phase downward, accentuated by downgaze and suppressed by upgaze | Craniocervical junction, e.g., tumor, malformation; cerebellar lesions |
| Horner's syndrome | Miosis and ptosis, often with ipsilateral hypohydrosis | Ipsilateral brain stem, spinal cord, lower brachial plexus, or cervical sympathetic chain |
| Left gaze preference | Eye looks left but may be driven across the midline by vestibulo-ocular reflexes | Left frontal lobe if preference can be overcome with doll's-head maneuver; right pons if not |
| Millard–Gubler syndrome | Ipsilateral CN VI and CN VII palsy and contralateral hemiparesis | Ipsilateral pons affecting the CN VI nucleus, intra-axial portion of CN VII, and corticospinal tract |
| Ocular bobbing | Jerking of eyes with a fast phase downward and slow return | Pons; some diffuse brain stem lesions may also produce ocular bobbing |
| Parinaud's syndrome | Impaired upward gaze with dilated and non-reactive pupils | Midbrain; usually compressive lesions, e.g., pineal tumor |
| Skew deviation | Vertical diplopia with one eye persistently elevated | Brain stem or cerebellum; lower eye is on side of the lesion |
| Internuclear ophthalmoplegia | Impaired adduction of contralateral eye with gaze to one side | Medial longitudinal fasciculus on side of eye that fails to adduct |
| Horizontal nystagmus | Fast deviation of eyes to one side with slower return to opposite side | Brain stem or vestibular system; many brain stem strokes and tumors are associated with horizontal nystagmus |

CN = cranial nerve.

PARIETAL AND OCCIPITAL LOBE LESIONS

The parieto-occipital cortex is involved in smooth pursuit—that is, in directing attention to an object of interest. Optic radiations project to the striate cortex of the occipital lobe; the prestriate region of the cortex is involved in analysis of this input. Lesions in this parieto-occipital region result in impaired pursuit movements in both directions of horizontal gaze in the contralateral visual field.

*Brain Stem Lesions*

Brain stem lesions that predominantly affect eye movements are discussed here, while those that produce other deficits are discussed in the brain stem section below. Some important entities affecting eye movements discussed later include Parinaud's syndrome, Millard–Gubler syndrome, and Foville's syndrome.

HORNER'S SYNDROME

Horner's syndrome consists of miosis (pupil constriction) plus ptosis and is a manifestation of damage to sympathetic fibers. Associated findings may include ipsilateral anhydrosis (impaired sweating), enophthalmos, and, in congenital cases, hypopigmentation of the iris. Although the pupil is small, it reacts normally to light and accommodation. Causes of Horner's syndrome include lesions at the following levels:

- Brain stem
- Spinal cord
- Brachial plexus
- Sympathetic chain

Brain stem lesions affect the sympathetic fibers as they descend into the spinal cord. The sympathetic pathway is adjacent to the spinothalamic tract, so Horner's syndrome due to a brain stem lesion is often associated with contralateral loss of pain and temperature sensation. Symptoms associated with specific brain stem syndromes are discussed below; many of them are associated with Horner's syndrome.

The sympathetic fibers descend in the lateral aspect of the cervical cord, and lesions in this region can produce Horner's syndrome.

Central cord lesions may produce bilateral Horner's syndrome, which is clinically difficult to recognize; ptosis and miosis with no other ocular motor abnormality suggest this syndrome.

The sympathetic efferents exit at T1; they briefly join the brachial plexus then ascend in the cervical sympathetic chain. Lesions affecting the T1 root may include intervertebral disk lesions, avulsion injuries, cervical rib lesions, and tumors.

The cervical sympathetic chain ascends with the carotid artery into the skull, through the cavernous sinus, then into the orbit. Lesions of these axons can occur with neck and skull-base tumors and carotid surgery. Lesions can also be found in the cavernous sinus and posterior aspect of the orbit.

Horner's syndrome may occur with cluster headache and occasionally migraine. Diagnosis is by typical history and exclusion of other causes.

INTERNUCLEAR OPHTHALMOPLEGIA
Internuclear ophthalmoplegia is characterized by a defect in adduction of one eye with lateral gaze. The abducting eye has nystagmus. The lesion is in the MLF in the brain stem, which connects the PPRF to the third nerve nuclear complex. The MLF crosses shortly after leaving the PPRF, so the lesion is ipsilateral to the eye that exhibits the difficulty with adduction.

Convergence is usually preserved in INO, and there are often no subjective complaints from the patient to suggest an ocular motor abnormality. Associated findings may include upward or torsional nystagmus and skew deviation.

Common causes of INO are multiple sclerosis and infarction. Because of the proximity of the MLF to the midline, INO is often bilateral.

ONE-AND-A-HALF SYNDROME
The one-and-a-half syndrome is a gaze palsy with an INO. It is due to a lesion in the pons affecting the PPRF, sixth nerve nucleus, and ipsilateral MLF. The only intact horizontal eye movement is abduc-

tion of the contralateral eye. The most common causes of this syndrome are multiple sclerosis and infarction.

SKEW DEVIATION

Skew deviation is characterized by vertical diplopia that cannot be explained by a cranial nerve palsy or extraocular muscle lesion. The lesion is in the brain stem or cerebellum. The most common cause of skew deviation is infarction. The lower eye is on the side of the lesion.

HORIZONTAL NYSTAGMUS

Horizontal nystagmus can be of central or peripheral origin. The differential diagnosis is aided by examination of the characteristics of the nystagmus. Vestibular dysfunction produces nystagmus with a slow component toward the side of the lesion. Gaze toward the side opposite the lesion accentuates the slow phase of the nystagmus.

Lesions of the brain stem commonly produce nystagmus. Nystagmus of central origin is differentiated from nystagmus of peripheral origin by several features:

- Central nystagmus is not suppressed by fixation whereas peripheral nystagmus is.
- Central nystagmus rarely has a torsional component whereas peripheral nystagmus commonly does.
- Latency to evoked nystagmus with the Báránay maneuvers is shorter with central lesions than with peripheral lesions (see Table 3.4).
- Duration of evoked nystagmus with the Báránay maneuvers is longer with central lesions than with peripheral lesions (see Table 3.4).

Nystagmus is common with many lesions of the brain stem, especially strokes and tumors; these are discussed below in the brain stem section. A few beats of nystagmus at extremes of gaze are considered normal and should not be confused with clearly abnormal movements.

**Table 3.4    Vertigo with Provocative Maneuvers**

| Clinical Finding | Peripheral Cause | Central Cause |
| --- | --- | --- |
| Latency | 0–40s | None |
| Duration | Brief, mean 7.8s | Long, may be persistent |
| Intensity | Severe | Mild to moderate |
| Nystagmus | Limited duration, consistent direction | Persistent, changing direction |
| Nausea with or without vomiting | Severe | Mild |

DOWNBEAT NYSTAGMUS

Downbeat nystagmus is evident in the primary position and is accentuated by downward gaze. Upward gaze suppresses the nystagmus. Lesion is classically at the cervicomedullary junction, although other brain stem lesions can produce this finding. The differential diagnosis is extensive and includes tumors, craniocervical subluxation, Arnold–Chiari malformation, basilar invagination, and hydrocephalus. Cerebellar degeneration can be associated with downbeat nystagmus in the absence of direct cervicomedullary pathology.

OCULAR BOBBING

Ocular bobbing is characterized by a rapid conjugate downgaze followed by a slower return to the primary position. The defect is usually bilateral. Lesion is of the pons and can be due to tumor, infarction, or hemorrhage within the substance; less frequently, extrinsic compressive lesions are found. Uncommon causes are encephalitis and central pontine myelinolysis. Inverse ocular bobbing, with the fast phase upward, is less likely to be due to a focal structural lesion and more likely to be due to anoxia or prolonged status epilepticus.

OCULOGYRIC CRISIS

Oculogyric crisis is an uncommonly recognized disorder characterized by spasmodic conjugate ocular deviations, usually upward and sometimes lateral. It is most commonly caused by neuroleptics, but it can also be seen with carbamazepine, lithium, and head injury. The patient can often voluntarily suppress the deviation, but only briefly.

*Individual Cranial Nerve Lesions*

CRANIAL NERVE III PALSY

Lesions of the third nerve are most common in the following locations:

- Intracranial segment near the posterior cerebral artery
- Intracranial segment near the tentorium cerebellum
- Intracranial segment, independent of a structural lesion
- Cavernous sinus
- Orbit

Proximity of the nerve to the posterior cerebral and posterior communicating arteries makes it susceptible to compression by aneurysms. This is the prime concern of clinicians when they observe a large, poorly reactive pupil.

The third nerve can be compressed by transtentorial herniation of the uncus with increased intracranial pressure. Fibers serving pupillary response may be affected before ocular movements because of their peripheral location on the nerve.

The third nerve is commonly damaged by ischemia as it passes through the subarachnoid space. Ischemia is seen with diabetes and hypertension, although neither may be present. Pupillary fibers may be spared because their peripheral location protects them from infarction by vessels penetrating the nerve. Therefore, pupil response is an important differentiating feature: early pupillary dilation favors a compressive lesion while a pupil-sparing third nerve palsy is more commonly ischemic. However, this is not an absolute differentiating feature, and pupil-sparing third nerve palsies with compressive lesions are not infrequent.

In the cavernous sinus, the third nerve is near the carotid artery and trochlear, abducens, and trigeminal nerves. There is a rostral–caudal anatomical organization as well, which influences the effect of lesions depending on whether they are nearer the orbit or the brain. Lesions that can affect the oculomotor nerve in the cavernous sinus include aneurysms, thrombophlebitis, and extension of nasopharyngeal tumors.

Lesion in the orbit can affect the superior and/or inferior divisions of the oculomotor nerve; in addition, it can interfere with movement of the globe because of mechanical effects. Pain and proptosis are common in this setting.

CRANIAL NERVE IV PALSY

Trochlear nerve palsy produces vertical diplopia plus head tilt to the side opposite the lesion; the head tilt compensates for diplopia due to extortion of the eye produced by the superior oblique palsy. The most common cause of fourth nerve palsy is trauma, which accounts for 34 percent of all cases; 20 percent of these are bilateral. Infarction of the nerve can occur in diabetes mellitus and atherosclerotic disease. Most other causes result in signs referable to midbrain or other cranial nerve(s). Other cranial neuropathies suggest a meningeal process. Involvement of CN III and/or VI suggests a lesion in the cavernous sinus or superior orbital fissure. Corticospinal tract signs or ataxia suggests a midbrain lesion.

CRANIAL NERVE VI PALSY

Abducens palsy can be due to lesion at almost any point from the nucleus to the distal nerve as it enters the lateral rectus in the orbit. Nuclear sixth lesions are more common than third or fourth nerve palsies. Because of the proximity to the PPRF and intra-axial portion of the facial nerve, conjugate gaze palsy and facial weakness often accompany the lateral rectus weakness. Lesion of the subarachnoid portion of the abducens nerve may develop from increased intracranial pressure, head injury, nerve infarction from diabetes or atherosclerotic disease, and meningitis.

*Extraocular Muscle Lesions*

Extraocular muscles may be affected directly by lesions, which must be differentiated from ocular motor nerve lesions. Careful examination reveals a pattern of weakness that cannot be explained by lesions of a single cranial nerve or combination of nerves. Common causes of extraocular muscle disease include the following:

- Trauma
- Thyroid ophthalmopathy
- Myasthenia gravis

Trauma can affect the ocular motor muscles by entrapment, which is common with orbital fractures. The defect may initially be missed because of periorbital edema, which impedes examination.

Thyroid ophthalmopathy is due to inflammation and fibrosis of ocular muscles. Exophthalmos is associated with this and usually precedes the ocular motor disorder. The most severely affected muscles include the inferior rectus, with the medial rectus, superior rectus, and obliques affected to a lesser extent.

Myasthenia gravis is associated with weakness of the ocular muscles that cannot be explained by single neural lesions. The medial rectus is commonly affected, but any muscle may be involved. Ptosis is common and is usually asymmetric. The defects are exacerbated by sustained gaze using affected muscles. Diagnosis is supported by improvement with edrophonium injection, although neurogenic lesions may show some improvement with this treatment as well.

*Pupillary Abnormalities*
The control of pupil diameter has been discussed, and pupillary abnormalities in relation to many lesions have also been presented. This section concerns problems that are confined to the pupil, with no other ocular motor abnormalities. Table 3.5 shows the anatomic correlates to pupillary abnormalities.

AFFERENT PUPIL (GUNN PUPIL)
An afferent pupillary defect is caused by a lesion of the optic nerve. The motor outflow to the pupils is normal, and the pupils are of equal size and react when the patient enters bright light. The defect is only evident when the eyes are tested individually. The swinging-flashlight test, discussed above, is particularly helpful in this diagnosis. With an afferent defect, the direct response is less prominent than the consensual response; as the light is alternated between eyes, illumination of the eye with the optic nerve lesions results in dilation of both pupils. In contrast, with partial third nerve lesions

**Table 3.5  Pupillary Abnormalities**

| Abnormality | Clinical Features | Localization |
|---|---|---|
| Anisocoria | Asymmetry in pupil diameter, but both respond normally | None |
| Argyll Robertson pupil | Pupils respond to accommodation but less so to light | Midbrain lesion, as seen in meningovascular syphilis, tumor, diabetes |
| Hippus | Spontaneous variation in pupil size with steady illumination | No pathological significance |
| Horner's syndrome | Miosis and ptosis | Ipsilateral sympathetic fibers anywhere from brain stem to spinal cord to cervical sympathetic chain |
| Afferent pupil | Direct response less than consensual response | Optic nerve |
| Tonic pupil | Slow constriction to light; light-near dissociation | Ciliary ganglion or short ciliary nerves, as in Adie's tonic pupil syndrome (with depressed tendon reflexes) |
| Fixed, dilated pupil | Dilated pupil without reaction to light or accommodation | Third nerve |

the pupil responds incompletely to direct or consensual stimulation, but the contralateral side responds normally.

The differential diagnosis of optic nerve lesions includes tumor, optic neuritis, and trauma. Retinal lesions can also produce an afferent defect, although the lesion is usually more severe and retinal abnormalities are often apparent on funduscopic examination.

ARGYLL ROBERTSON PUPIL

The Argyll Robertson pupil is small, irregular, and unresponsive to light, although it responds to accommodation. The Argyll Robertson pupil is seen classically in meningovascular syphilis, but it can also be seen with tumors compressing the dorsal midbrain (such as pinealomas), diabetes, brain stem encephalitis, sarcoidosis, Adie's syndrome, amyloidosis, and glaucoma. The disparity between the responses to light and accommodation is probably due to a difference in the pathways involved in the reflexes.

TONIC PUPIL

Tonic pupil is dilated at rest and does not react to flashes of light. With sustained bright light, the pupil slowly constricts, and it does not immediately dilate on discontinuation of the light. Accommodation results in better constriction than light does, since accommodation is a stronger physiological stimulus for constriction.

The lesion with tonic pupil is usually of the ciliary ganglion or nerves from the ganglion to the eye. The disorder can be idiopathic (Adie's syndrome) or due to trauma or local orbital lesions (tumor, infection); it can also be a manifestation of peripheral neuropathy with autonomic symptoms.

OCULOMOTOR APRAXIA

Oculomotor apraxia is the inability to make voluntary saccades when the basic mechanisms for eye movements are intact. Reflexive eye movements are intact. Oculomotor apraxia can be congenital or acquired.

Congenital oculomotor apraxia presents in childhood with thrusting head movements during which the eyes close; this movement compensates for the saccadic deficit. Other neurologic deficits are frequently seen, including strabismus and developmental delay.

Acquired oculomotor apraxia can develop in patients with bilateral parietal damage and may be a manifestation of diffuse cerebral disease, such as hypoxic–ischemic encephalopathy. Patients may manifest some of the same head thrusting as seen in children with congenital oculomotor apraxia, but it is less marked.

**Trigeminal Nerve**

*Anatomy*

The trigeminal nerve exits the pons and travels anteriorly into Meckel's cavity where the sensory neuron cell bodies form the trigeminal ganglion. After the nerve fibers exit the ganglion, they divide into the ophthalmic (CN V1), maxillary (CN V2), and mandibular (CN V3) divisions.

The ophthalmic division (CN V1) travels through the cavernous sinus and enters the orbit through the superior orbital fissure. In the cavernous sinus, CN V1 is in proximity to CNs III, IV, and VI and also to CN V2 in the posterior aspect of the cavernous sinus. The ophthalmic division has no motor function; sensory function is to the forehead and scalp forward of the vertex, upper eyelid, upper aspect of the cornea, much of the nasal cavity, and lacrimal glands.

The maxillary division (CN V2) travels through the posterior aspect of the cavernous sinus, exits the skull via the foramen rotundum, and enters the orbit through the inferior orbital fissure. It then passes beneath the globe and exits onto the face via the infraorbital foramen. There is no motor function. The maxillary division provides sensation to the nose, upper lip, cheek, and lower half of cornea and conjunctiva. The maxillary sinus, upper teeth and gums, palate, and lower aspect of the nasal cavity are also supplied by this division.

The mandibular division (CN V3) is joined by the small motor fascicle of the trigeminal nerve and exits the skull via the foramen ovale. Motor supply is to the masseter, temporalis, ptergyoids, tensor tympani, and mylohyoid muscles. Sensory innervation is to the lower lip, chin, floor of the mouth, lower jaw and gums, and anterior tongue.

*Lesions*

The trigeminal nerve can be damaged in the posterior fossa intraaxially by tumors, vascular disease, vascular malformations, or demyelinating disease. Extra-axial involvement can be by tumor or vascular structures. Isolated lesions of the trigeminal nerve are unusual; the most common disorder is trigeminal neuralgia. Trigeminal nerve fibers can be affected by disorders affecting other neural elements, discussed elsewhere; some of the most important are the lateral medullary syndrome and lateral pontine syndrome.

*Trigeminal Neuralgia*

Trigeminal neuralgia is characterized by unilateral paroxysms of pain on the face. The pain is usually lancinating and follows one of the trigeminal divisions. Occasionally, the pain follows more than one division.

The localization of the lesion with trigeminal neuralgia is usually not determined; the patient's history strongly suggests the diagnosis. Examination is normal, although some patients report subjective sensory loss in the affected distribution. Trigeminal neuralgia is, therefore, usually considered idiopathic, although it may be seen in patients with vascular compression of the gasserian ganglion, demyelinating disease, and tumors with compression.

*Zoster of the Trigeminal Ganglion*

Zoster of the trigeminal ganglion, which is uncommon, can result in severe pain and paresthesia in the distribution of the trigeminal nerve. In contrast to trigeminal neuralgia, with zoster real sensory loss can occur.

*Raeder's Paratrigeminal Neuralgia*

This rare condition is characterized by pain in a trigeminal distribution with ipsilateral ptosis and miosis. Associated findings may include fourth or sixth nerve palsies. This condition is usually due to lesions in the vicinity of the trigeminal ganglion, including tumors, infections, and vascular malformations.

**Facial Nerve**

The facial nerve is the predominant supply of innervation to muscles of the face, but the nerve also has other functions. Precise documentation of affected functions can accurately localize a lesion; this localization depends on accurate knowledge of facial nerve anatomy.

### Anatomy

The facial motor nucleus is in the caudal pons. Efferent fibers arc dorsally around the abducens nucleus, then exit the ventral surface of the brain stem. The motor nerve is joined by fibers from the superior salivatory nucleus and nucleus of the solitary tract; it then joins CN VIII in the internal auditory canal (IAC). The facial nerve enters the facial canal at the terminus of the IAC. The nerve extends into the geniculate ganglion, which contains cell bodies of fibers in the nervus intermedius. The nerve leaves the geniculate ganglion and travels toward the middle ear, where it gives rise to the nerve to the stapedius muscle and the chorda tympani. The facial nerve then passes through the stylomastoid foramen to the face. The posterior auricular nerve separates from the facial nerve near the stylomastoid foramen. The main trunk of the facial nerve passes through the parotid and divides into several named branches.

The chorda tympani carries taste from the anterior two thirds of the tongue to the nucleus of the solitary tract. Also, it carries the preganglionic parasympathetic fibers innervating the submandibular and sublingual glands.

The nervus intermedius carries the taste afferents and parasympathetic efferents that compose the chorda tympani, plus cutaneous afferents from the pinna, mastoid region, and external auditory canal (EAC). It also contains mucosal afferents from the nose, palate, and pharynx. These neurons have their cell bodies in the geniculate ganglion.

### Lesions

The most important differentiation for facial nerve dysfunction is between a central and a peripheral lesion. Because of the long and circuitous route of the facial nerve within the pons, brain stem lesions may produce what appears to be peripheral facial palsy. Table 3.6 lists findings with central and peripheral lesions that produce facial weakness.

Peripheral facial weakness is differentiated from central weakness by distribution and associated findings. The entire face is affected with peripheral lesions, while the lower face is predomi-

**Table 3.6 Facial Weakness**

| Lesion Location | Findings |
| --- | --- |
| Cerebral cortex | Lower face weakness, usually with arm weakness |
| Internal capsule | Lower facial weakness, usually with arm and leg weakness |
| Pons | Ipsilateral facial weakness, contralateral hemiparesis, ipsilateral appendicular ataxia |
| Subarachnoid space | Upper and lower face weakness without taste change |
| Internal auditory canal | Upper and lower face weakness; deafness and/or tinnitus if auditory portion of nerve is involved; loss of taste on anterior two thirds of tongue; hyperacusis |
| Geniculate ganglion | Upper and lower facial weakness with pain behind ear, and loss of taste on anterior two thirds of tongue; hyperacusis |
| Facial canal | Upper and lower facial weakness with loss of taste on anterior two thirds of tongue; hyperacusis |
| Below stylo-mastoid foramen | Upper and lower facial weakness; no other symptoms; if the division to the lower face is predominantly affected, findings may seem to indicate central lesion |

nantly affected with central lesions. This difference occurs because supranuclear input to the facial nuclei is bilateral for neurons controlling the upper face and mainly contralateral for neurons controlling the lower face.

Lesion of the facial nerve within the brain stem is usually associated with other neurologic findings, such as sixth nerve palsy or contralateral weakness; these findings in conjunction with a peripheral seventh palsy suggest a lesion in the caudal pons. Cerebral lesions producing lower facial weakness usually do not cause other brain stem signs and commonly produce arm weakness or incoordination ipsilateral to the facial palsy. Weakness contralateral to the facial palsy suggests a pontine lesion on the side of the facial weakness.

*Bell's Palsy*

Bell's palsy is idiopathic facial palsy with no other cranial neuropathies. The cause is not completely known, although some individuals believe that it can be due to zoster. Isolated facial palsy can be the first sign of Guillain–Barré syndrome.

The onset of idiopathic facial palsy is usually heralded by pain around and posterior to the ear, followed by weakness of the upper and lower face that may progress over several days. Associated symptoms may include hyperacusis and/or loss of taste over the ipsilateral anterior two thirds of the tongue, depending on the location of the lesion. Hyperacusis is an apparent increase in sound volume perceived by the ipsilateral ear. It is due to damage to the nerve to the stapedius, which arises from the facial nerve in the facial canal.

Peripheral facial nerve palsy is differentiated from a central lesion by involvement of the upper as well as the lower face; central lesions mostly affect the lower face. Brain stem lesions usually produce dysfunction of other cranial nerves or brain stem structures. Lacrimation is affected if the facial nerve lesion is proximal to the greater petrosal nerve.

*Ramsay Hunt Syndrome*

Ramsay Hunt syndrome in this context refers to zoster of the geniculate ganglion. The other disorder of the same name is a syndrome characterized by cerebellar ataxia plus myoclonus (discussed later in this chapter). Patients present with severe ear pain and usually have a vesicular eruption in the external auditory canal. The facial palsy usually follows the onset of pain by one to three days.

Diagnosis is confused if the vesicles are not observed or are attributed to otitis externa. A typical history of ear pain with "otitis externa" followed by facial weakness suggests Ramsay Hunt syndrome.

Occasionally, other cranial nerves may be affected, including the trigeminal and glossopharyngeal nerves. Sensory loss on the face and palate are symptoms associated with these lesions, respectively.

*Hemifacial Spasm*

Hemifacial spasm is an episodic clonic activity of one side of the face. It often begins in the region of the orbicularis oculi and then spreads to surrounding muscles innervated by the facial nerve. The location of the lesion is thought to be the facial nerve, since hemifacial spasm can occur after Bell's palsy, with tumors affecting the facial nerve, or following local facial trauma. Some patients develop hemifacial spasm due to pulsation of a small artery against the facial nerve.

## Vestibulocochlear Nerve

*Anatomy*

The eighth nerve serves sensory function from the vestibular apparatus and cochlea. The vestibular apparatus consists of three semicircular canals organized roughly orthogonally in the x, y, and z planes, and the semicircular canals detect head rotation in these planes. In addition, there are organs that sense head tilt and horizontal acceleration (utricle) and vertical acceleration (saccule). Deformation of cellular processes (kinocilia) produces activation of the cells in the vestibulocochlear nerve.

The cochlea transduces auditory input into action potentials in the eighth nerve. Vibration in the air creates vibration of the tympanic membrane; the vibration is then conducted mechanically to the ossicles and cochlea through the oval window, which in turn sets up vibration in the perilymph and basilar membrane. Hair cells have their bodies on the basilar membrane, while the hairs project into the tectorial membrane. The basilar membrane is organized through its length so that high frequencies are transduced near the oval window and low frequencies are transduced near the apex.

Output from the vestibular apparatus and cochlea is conducted in the eighth nerve through the internal auditory canal to the brain stem where fibers from the cochlea project to the cochlear nuclei. Efferents from the cochlear nuclei cross and ascend in the contralateral lateral lemniscus. Some project to the superior olivary complex, others to the reticular formation bilaterally. Ascending fibers terminate in the inferior colliculus, which in turn projects to the medial geniculate. Efferents from the medial geniculate ascend to the primary auditory cortex, area 41, on the temporal lobe (discussed later in this chapter). Throughout much of this pathway, the auditory projections are organized tonotopically—that is, they are spatially arranged according to frequency.

Vestibular outflow enters the brain stem and terminates in the vestibular nuclei, which are actually a complex of nuclei. Vestibular input is used by several systems, including the cerebellum for error correction during movement, the spinal cord for control over antigravity muscles, and the eye movement control mechanisms.

## *Lesions*

Lesions of the eighth nerve can affect one or both sensory modalities—that is, vestibular and cochlear. Vestibular dysfunction causes vertigo, nausea and vomiting, and imbalanced walking; nystagmus is found on examination with no objective signs of brain stem dysfunction. Auditory dysfunction presents with hearing loss and often tinnitus, which is frequently the earliest sign of eighth nerve dysfunction.

Differentiation between a brain stem lesion and a vestibulocochlear nerve lesion can be difficult. Both can present with the nonspecific complaint of dizziness, which may mean vertigo, presyncope, ataxia, orthostasis, panic—attack response, and/or other vague disorders. Vertigo, a perception of movement of the patient or environment, is the relevant finding. Table 3.4 lists the responses to Báránay maneuvers with central and peripheral lesions producing vertigo. A vestibulocochlear nerve lesion is suggested by the following findings:

- Latency of several seconds between head movement and symptoms
- Symptoms lasting less than one minute
- Fatigue with repetitive provocation

- Severe vertigo, often with nausea and vomiting, which may be incapacitating
- No associated signs of brain stem dysfunction

A brain stem lesion is suggested by the following findings:

- Immediate onset of symptoms after head movement
- Long-lasting and/or persistent symptoms after head movement
- Frequent lack of fatigue with repetitive provocation
- Mild to moderate sensation of vertigo
- Often other associated signs of brain stem dysfunction

Ataxia of gait is common with central and peripheral disorders, but patients with peripheral disorders usually have good coordination of individual limbs.

*Acoustic Neuroma*
Acoustic neuroma is a schwannoma of the vestibular portion of the eighth nerve. Common presenting symptoms include tinnitus and hearing loss. Pressure on surrounding structures can produce ataxia, facial pain (from trigeminal involvement), facial weakness (from facial nerve involvement), and other brain stem signs (from direct compression). Despite the vestibular branch origin, vertigo is uncommon.

Confirmation of diagnosis requires MRI with special attention to the IAC and cerebellopontine angle. Brain stem auditory evoked potentials are helpful.

*Benign Positional Vertigo*
Benign positional vertigo is characterized by paroxysms of vertigo triggered by a certain position or certain direction of head movement. Table 3.4 presents guidelines for differentiating between central and peripheral vertigo.

*Peripheral Vestibulopathy*
Peripheral vestibulopathy encompasses the diagnoses of vestibular neuronitis and labyrinthitis; while some experts make a distinction between the two, in practice, this differentiation is blurred. Patients present with episodes of vertigo interspersed with periods without

neurologic symptoms. Peripheral vestibulopathy is differentiated from benign positional vertigo by the absence of a precise positional component. Many patients seek medical attention with their first episode, which may lead to concern over other possibilities, including brain stem infarction, tumor, and demyelinating disease.

### Meniere's Disease

Meniere's disease is characterized by attacks of vertigo associated with a roaring sound. The attacks abate within a day or so but are followed by hearing loss. The auditory symptoms are key to the diagnosis.

### Multiple Sclerosis

Dizziness is a common early symptom in MS. The key to diagnosis is evidence of other neurologic lesions on history and examination. In practice, the diagnosis is rarely made at the first encounter. The dizziness may be a vague dysequilibrium or true vertigo.

Diagnosis depends on documentation of multiple lesions in space and time. MRI shows areas of increased signal intensity in the white matter on T2-weighted images. Cerebrospinal fluid studies can be supportive.

## Glossopharyngeal Nerve

### Anatomy

The ninth nerve exits from the brain stem in the medulla and then exits the cranial vault through the jugular foramen. Subsequently it nears the carotid artery and jugular vein and terminates in the pharynx.

The ninth nerve supplies the stylopharyngeus muscle and, in conjunction with the tenth, the constrictors of the pharynx. Sources of sensory supply include the posterior pharynx, soft palate, tonsillar pillars, posterior nasopharynx, and posterior one third of the tongue. The ninth nerve also carries taste from the posterior third of the tongue. The sensory fiber cell bodies are in the petrous ganglion in the distal aspect of the jugular foramen.

### Lesions

Lesions of the ninth nerve are unusual and difficult to identify. The stylopharyngeus muscle cannot be tested by routine examination. The gag and palatal reflexes use ninth nerve afferents but the efferents are vagal.

### Glossopharyngeal Neuralgia

Glossopharyngeal neuralgia is a rare condition characterized by severe lancinating pain in the posterior pharynx, usually in the region of the tonsils. It is occasionally associated with syncope, which is attributed to activation of carotid sinus afferents. Glossopharyngeal neuralgia is usually idiopathic, but structural lesions must be considered, including tumors and vascular malformations at the cerebellopontine angle.

### Nasopharyngeal Lesions

Nasopharyngeal lesions may produce glossopharyngeal deficits in conjunction with lesions of any or all of CNs X, XI, and XII. The most common pathology is probably neoplastic, but infections, trauma, and postoperative deficits account for many of these cases.

### Glomus Jugulare Tumors

Glomus jugulare tumors arise from the chemoreceptors of the jugular bulb. They can present with ninth nerve deficits, including impaired gag reflex. Typical symptoms include pulsatile tinnitus and hearing loss from CN VIII involvement. The patient may have headaches due to increased intracranial pressure, which is associated with obstruction of jugular vein outflow. Erosion of surrounding bone and vascularization may produce a pulsatile vascular structure in the EAC. Accessory nerve involvement may produce sternocleidomastoid and trapezius weakness. Vagal involvement may produce dysphonia and signs of vocal cord paralysis.

## Vagus

### Anatomy

The dorsal motor nucleus of the vagus sits on the floor of the fourth ventricle in the brain stem. It gives rise to preganglionic parasympathetic fibers that have widespread projections from the pharynx to thoracic and abdominal organs. The nucleus ambiguus in the medullary reticular formation supplies all of the striated muscles of the pharynx and larynx innervated by the vagus.

Vagal afferents serving general visceral sensation from the pharynx, larynx, and thoracic and abdominal organs terminate in the nucleus solitarius and have their cell bodies in the nodose ganglion. Vagal afferents serving taste from the posterior pharynx also terminate in the nucleus solitarius with cell bodies in the nodose ganglion. Vagal afferents serving sensation from the ear terminate in the spinal tract of CN V and have their cell bodies in the jugular ganglion.

The vagus exits the brain stem in the lateral medulla, near the exit of the glossopharyngeal nerve. It exits the skull via the jugular foramen, after which it divides into functionally distinct divisions: the auricular ramus supplies skin of the external ear; the meningeal ramus supplies some of the dura intracranially; and the pharyngeal ramus innervates muscles of the pharynx and soft palate, the superior laryngeal nerve (which serves as a motor to the cricothyroid and sensory input to the larynx), and the vagal nerve.

The vagal nerve descends in the neck and has branches supplying the heart (cardiac rami) and recurrent laryngeal nerves. The recurrent laryngeal nerves innervate the vocal cords but take different paths through the chest; the left passes beneath the aortic arch, and the right moves past the subclavian artery. Together they innervate most of the muscles of the larynx. The right and left vagal nerves descend through the mediastinum and enter the abdomen through the esophageal opening in the diaphragm. The vagal divisions innervate the large and small intestine, stomach, pancreas, and liver.

### Lesions

Isolated lesion of the whole vagus is uncommon. Several brain stem syndromes may result in vagal dysfunction; they are presented at the end of this chapter.

*Recurrent Laryngeal Nerve Palsy*

This is the most commonly diagnosed vagal dysfunction in clinical practice and should be a flag of chest pathology. Patients present with hoarseness, which may be initially attributed to bronchitis or sinusitis. However, the persistence of the hoarseness leads to further medical evaluation. Laryngoscopy reveals unilateral vocal cord paralysis. Chest x-ray or computerized tomography confirms the diagnosis. Common causes of recurrent laryngeal nerve palsy include tumors affecting the mediastinum and aneurysms of the subclavian artery or aortic arch. No cause is identified in some patients.

Vincristine has been implicated in some cases of unilateral recurrent laryngeal nerve palsy, although infiltration by the cancer for which the patient was given the drug has to be ruled out. Peripheral neuropathy uncommonly affects vagal nerves, but when it does, it produces bilateral deficits.

*Pseudobulbar Palsy*

Pseudobulbar palsy is impairment of bulbar function due to bilateral supranuclear lesions. Bilateral lesions are required for this palsy to be seen because of the bilateral descending innervation of the motor nuclei. Bifrontal infarctions or contusions are common causes of pseudobulbar palsy, although the differential diagnosis is huge. Patients present with dysphagia and dysarthria. Associated features unrelated to brain stem function include emotional volatility with uncontrollable and often inappropriate laughing and crying.

## Accessory Nerve

### *Anatomy*

The accessory nerve is composed of motor axons that originate in the nucleus ambiguus of the medulla and the accessory nucleus in the cervical spinal cord. The accessory nucleus is an elongated column of cells that extends from spinal levels C1 to C5. Neurons from C1 and C2 mainly innervate the sternocleidomastoid, while neurons from C3 and C4 mostly innervate the trapezius.

Small rootlets exit the medulla and brain stem at multiple levels and join to form the accessory nerve, which exits the skull via the jugular foramen. The most prominent function of the accessory nerve is innervation of the sternocleidomastoid and trapezius muscles. The axons from the nucleus ambiguus form separately from the main trunk of the accessory nerve to join the vagus in innervating muscles of the pharynx and larynx.

Supranuclear innervation of the muscles is somewhat uncertain, but it is believed that the motoneurons to the trapezius receive predominantly crossed upper motoneuron innervation while the neurons to the sternocleidomastoid receive bilateral upper motoneuron innervation.

### Lesions

Pure lesions of the accessory nerve are unusual in clinical practice; when present, they are usually due to local tumor infiltration or surgery. Catheterization of the internal jugular has been reported as a cause. Accessory nerve damage results in weakness of the ipsilateral sternocleidomastoid and trapezius. The ipsilateral sternocleidomastoid weakness causes impaired turning toward the side opposite the lesion. Many causes of accessory palsy also cause dysfunction of other cranial nerves; they are discussed at the end of this chapter.

## Hypoglossal Nerve

### Anatomy

The hypoglossal nucleus is on the floor of the fourth ventricle and contains the motoneurons that innervate the tongue. The nucleus is elongated, and multiple rootlets exit along a line between the pyramid and olive of the medulla. The rootlets converge to form the hypoglossal nerve, which exits the skull via the hypoglossal canal.

The hypoglossal nerve travels through the neck, passing near the internal carotid artery, to the base of the tongue where it divides into multiple branches. The hypoglossal nerve supplies innervation to the tongue and the genioglossus and geniohyoid muscles.

### Lesions

*Hypoglossal Nerve Lesions*
Isolated lesion of the hypoglossal nerve is uncommon; usually, multiple lower cranial nerves are affected. These syndromes are discussed below.

Lesion of the hypoglossal nerve results in impaired movement of the tongue, with resultant dysarthria and dysphagia. The tongue deviates to the side of the lesion because of impaired protrusion. Neck injuries, tumors, and infections can result in unilateral hypoglossal lesions with only partial paralysis of the tongue.

*Supranuclear Lesions*
Supranuclear lesions have little effect on many pharyngeal muscles unless the lesions are bilateral. However, unilateral corticobulbar lesion can result in deviation of the tongue, which protrudes toward the side of the hemiparesis. Supranuclear lesions are differentiated from nuclear and nerve lesions by the absence of atrophy on examination and the absence of denervation on electromyography (EMG).

## BRAIN STEM

Brain stem anatomy includes associated connections with the cerebellum, spinal cord, and hemispheres. In addition, cranial nerve anatomy and function are integral to brain stem anatomy. Clinical diagnosis of brain stem dysfunction requires understanding of motor and sensory pathways through the brain stem and a working knowledge of segmental anatomy at different levels of the brain stem. Table 3.7 presents the localization and clinical features of some important brain stem syndromes.

### Overview

Remembering the segmental anatomy of the brain stem is easier if sites of exit of the cranial nerves are thoroughly understood. Figure 3.1 shows a ventral view of the brain stem with sites of exit of each cranial nerve, and Figure 3.2 shows the vascular supply of the brain stem.

**Table 3.7    Brain Stem Syndromes**

| Syndrome | Structures Affected | Features |
|---|---|---|
| *Midbrain* | | |
| Parinaud's syndrome | Dorsal midbrain, pretectal region, posterior commissure | Vertical gaze deficit, usually supranuclear; light-near dissociation of pupil response; convergence–retraction nystagmus; lid retraction; lid lag |
| Weber's syndrome | CN III, ventral midbrain, corticospinal tract | CN III palsy, contralateral hemiparesis |
| Syndrome of Benedikt | CN III, ventral midbrain, corticospinal tract, red nucleus | CN III palsy, contralateral hemiparesis, intention tremor, cerebellar ataxia |
| Top-of-the-basilar syndrome | Occipital lobes, midbrain ocular motor nuclei, cerebral peduncle, medial temporal lobe, thalamus | Cortical blindness, ocular motor defects, corticospinal signs, memory deficit, sensory deficits |
| *Pons* | | |
| Millard–Gubler syndrome | CN VI, CN VII, ventral pons | CN VI and VII palsies, contralateral hemiparesis |
| Clumsy hand–dysarthria syndrome | Corticospinal tract, facial nerve | Hemiparesis, dysarthria, often with facial weakness |
| Locked-in syndrome | Corticospinal tracts, facial nerves, abducens nerve | Quadriplegia, facial weakness, lateral gaze palsy |
| Pure motor hemiparesis: pons | Corticospinal tract in the ventral pons | Hemiparesis with corticospinal tract signs; no other neurologic signs |
| Ataxic hemiparesis: pons | Corticospinal tract at basis pontis (or internal capsule of cerebrum) | Hemiparesis with impaired coordination |

**Table 3.7 (*continued*)**

| Syndrome | Structures Affected | Features |
|---|---|---|
| Foville syndrome | CN VII, ventral pons, PPRF | CN VII palsy, contralateral hemiparesis, gaze palsy to side of lesion |
| ***Medulla*** | | |
| Lateral medullary syndrome (Wallenberg's syndrome) | Inferior cerebellar peduncle, descending sympathetic tract, spinothalamic tract, trigeminal nucleus | Ipsilateral ataxia, Horner's syndrome, vertigo, contralateral pain and temperature loss, ipsilateral facial sensory loss |
| Medial medullary syndrome (Dejerine's syndrome) | Corticospinal tract, medial lemniscus, hypoglossal nerve | Contralateral hemiparesis; loss of position and vibratory sensation; ipsilateral tongue paresis |

CN = cranial nerve; PPRF = paramedian pontine reticular formation.

The oculomotor nerve exits the midbrain on the ventral surface between the cerebral peduncles. The trochlear nerve exits the midbrain near the inferior colliculus and wraps around the cerebral peduncle. The optic nerve only projects a small proportion of its fibers to the midbrain, but the optic tracts sit just above the oculomotor and trochlear nerves as they travel toward the orbit.

Immediately below the midbrain is the pons, which on ventral view appears to wrap around the brain stem and attach to the cerebellar hemispheres on either side. The trigeminal nerve exits the lateral aspect of the pons.

The abducens, facial, and vestibulocochlear nerves exit at the pontomedullary junction. The most medial is the abducens nerve, which has a long course past the pons to project to the orbit. The facial nerve exits laterally to the abducens and just adjacent to the vestibulocochlear nerve. The glossopharyngeal, vagus, and hypoglos-

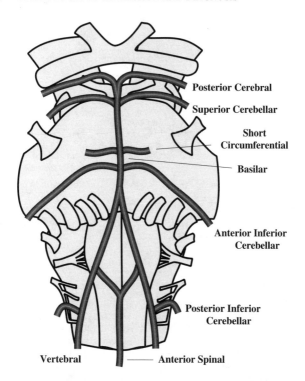

**Fig. 3.2** Shown are the arterial supply of the brain stem and its relationship to posterior fossa structures.

sal nerves exit the medulla, and the accessory nerve has fibers that exit at both the level of the medulla and the upper cervical cord.

Localization of lesions affecting the brain stem is easier if a systematic approach is used. When faced with a difficult diagnostic problem, I try to rely on this method rather than blindly trying to fit the symptoms into one of the very many syndrome descriptions. Important questions to answer include the following:

1. Is the lesion intra-axial or extra-axial?
2. What is the rostral–caudal location of the lesion?
3. Is the intra-axial lesion unilateral or bilateral?
4. What clinical conditions can produce damage in this localization?

Isolated single cranial nerve palsies are usually extra-axial—that is, not in the substance of the brain stem. Multiple cranial nerve palsies can still be due to extra-axial disease. An intra-axial lesion is suggested by the combination of cranial nerve palsies and signs of damage to ascending and descending tracts. For example, an isolated CN VI palsy, which causes defective abduction of the ipsilateral eye, is relatively common and can result from microvascular disease, trauma, and increased intracranial pressure; it is often idiopathic. In contrast, a CN VI palsy combined with damage to the medial longitudinal fasciculus, which causes internuclear ophthalmoplegia, is due to a lesion in the pons.

Rostral–caudal localization is most easily identified by carefully determining which cranial nerves are affected. For example, an oculomotor lesion with signs of intra-axial damage suggests a midbrain lesion, while glossopharyngeal and vagus damage suggests a medullary lesion.

Determination of whether the lesion is unilateral or bilateral requires understanding of which tracts are crossed and at which level. The descending corticospinal tracts cross in the medulla. Dorsal column axons—which serve touch, vibration, and position sense—ascend the cord uncrossed, synapse in the nucleus gracilis and nucleus cuneatus in the medulla, and cross as they ascend through the medulla, forming the medial lemniscus. The spinothalamic tract axons, which convey pain and temperature sensations, cross at the level of the spinal cord segment and ascend crossed in the cord. The spinothalamic tract stays lateral in the brain stem and ascends to the midbrain where it joins with the medial lemniscus to enter the thalamus.

Once the lesion has been determined to be intra-axial and the rostral–caudal and unilateral or bilateral localization has been made, individual syndromes can be considered. Specific etiologies are suggested by associated symptoms; for instance, acute onset of a deficit suggests a stroke, sudden onset of headache and vomiting suggests a hemorrhage, and a slowly progressive deficit suggests an expanding mass lesion.

### Midbrain

#### *Anatomy*

Figure 3.3 shows a cross-section of the midbrain between the superior and inferior colliculi. Important landmarks are the cerebral peduncles, red nucleus, substantia nigra, aqueduct and surrounding periaqueductal gray matter, medial lemniscus, medial longitudinal fasciculus, and midbrain tectum.

The cerebral peduncles carry descending information from the cerebral hemispheres to the brain stem and spinal cord. The red nucleus receives outflow from the contralateral cerebellum and sends efferents to the thalamus. The medial lemniscus carries ascending fibers from the nucleus gracilis and nucleus cuneatus in the medulla to the thalamus. The substantia nigra has extensive interconnections with other nuclei, but the most important are the reciprocal connections with the striatum.

The oculomotor nuclear complex is adjacent to the midline and ventral to the aqueduct. The trochlear nucleus is in a similar position, but it is caudal to the oculomotor nucleus, although still within the midbrain. The medial longitudinal fasciculus carries outflow from the contralateral paramedial pontine reticular formation, the center of which governs lateral gaze, and projects to the oculomotor nuclear complex.

Blood supply to the midbrain is largely through the basilar artery, which lies on the ventral surface. The basilar artery sends sev-

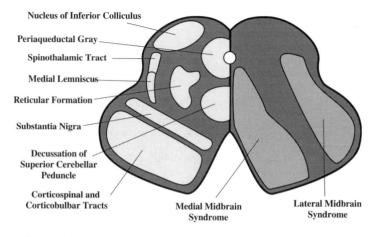

**Fig. 3.3**  Cross-section of the midbrain.

eral penetrating branches into the midbrain before bifurcating into the posterior cerebral arteries (PCAs), which wrap laterally around the midbrain. The PCAs also give off penetrating branches.

### Lesions

Isolated CN III or CN IV palsy is rarely due to a midbrain lesion, despite the location of the nuclei. Midbrain lesions can produce partial or complete palsies of these cranial nerves plus hemiparesis from involvement of the cerebral peduncle or ataxia from damage to the red nucleus. In addition to these direct effects of midbrain lesions, many such lesions can obstruct the aqueduct, producing hydrocephalus affecting the lateral and third but sparing the fourth ventricle.

Important lesions of the midbrain include infarctions, intrinsic tumors, and extrinsic compression by tumors in the pineal region. Some of these are discussed below. Basilar thrombosis and top-of-the-basilar syndrome affect the midbrain, but they affect other structures as well, so they are discussed at the end of this chapter.

*Parinaud's Syndrome*
Parinaud's syndrome is due to dysfunction of the rostral aspect of the dorsal midbrain. The most common cause is a tumor in the pineal region, but infarction or hemorrhage can also cause the syndrome. Hydrocephalus can produce downward displacement of tissue in the midbrain region, also producing Parinaud's syndrome. The lesion affects the pretectal region of the midbrain, the posterior commissure, and the interstitial nucleus.

Patients present with supranuclear difficulty with vertical gaze—that is, there is defective voluntary gaze but preserved vertical vestibulo-ocular reflexes. Pupillary response is impaired to light but relatively preserved to accommodation (light-near dissociation). Other classic findings are convergence–retraction nystagmus, lid retraction, and lid lag. Convergence–retraction nystagmus consists of rhythmic convergence and divergence movements induced by upward gaze.

Partial lesions are often seen, making identification of the entire clinical syndrome uncommon. In practice, defective vertical gaze with light-near dissociation, often with unequal pupils, suggests the lesion. Since many patients with this syndrome have tumors, extension into the hypothalamic region can produce diabetes insipidus. Lesion of the caudal midbrain at the level of the inferior colliculus can produce defective downward gaze with preservation of pupillary responses.

*Weber's Syndrome*
Weber's syndrome is contralateral hemiparesis with ipsilateral oculomotor palsy that does not spare the pupil. It is due to damage to the cerebral peduncle and oculomotor nerve. The most common

cause is posterior circulation ischemia, although tumors can produce the symptoms.

*Syndrome of Benedikt*
The syndrome of Benedikt consists of contralateral hemiparesis, ipsilateral oculomotor palsy, and contralateral cerebellar ataxia. The ataxia is a combination of corticospinal dysfunction and damage to the red nucleus.

## Pons

### Anatomy

Figure 3.4 shows a cross section of the pons. There are rostral–caudal differences in organization, so this figure is slightly stylized

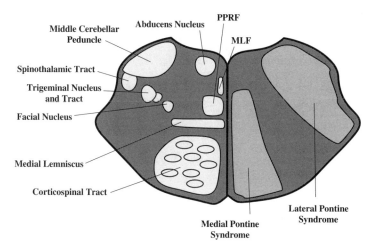

**Fig. 3.4** Cross-section of the pons.

to show important structures. Important landmarks include the corticospinal tract, pontine nuclei, medial lemniscus, spinothalamic tract, lateral lemniscus, nuclei and intra-axial portions of the abducens, trigeminal and facial nerves, vestibular nucleus, PPRF, and MLF.

The corticospinal tract lies in the ventral aspect of the pons, and it is still uncrossed at this level. The medial lemniscus, carrying fibers from the nuclei gracilis and cuneatus, is already crossed. The PPRF, which is important for lateral gaze, sends output to the abducens nucleus and through the MLF to the midbrain. The MLF is not dedicated solely to the PPRF, however; it also carries descending axons of the medial reticulospinal and vestibulospinal tracts and the tectospinal tract. The motor and sensory nuclei of the trigeminal nerves lie rostral to the abducens and facial nuclei, which lie in the posterior half of the pons. The facial nerve exits the facial nucleus and moves dorsally to loop around the abducens nucleus before moving ventrally and medially to exit the brain stem at the pontomedullary junction.

The vertebral arteries join to form the basilar artery near the pontomedullary junction, and basilar artery ascends to the midbrain. There are major and minor circumferential branches as well as direct penetrating paramedial branches of the basilar artery. Major circumferential branches include the anterior inferior cerebellar artery (AICA) and superior cerebellar arteries. Transverse arteries have a variable projection bilaterally and send penetrating arteries into the pons.

*Lesions*

Pontine lesions can produce varied lesions depending on the rostral–caudal and dorsal–ventral extent of the damage. Important symptoms suggesting a pontine lesion include lateral gaze palsy from PPRF dysfunction, facial or abducens nerve palsy, signs of parenchymal damage, such as corticospinal tract dysfunction.

Lesions of the pons that produce predominantly ocular motor abnormalities were discussed earlier in the section on cranial nerves.

*Millard–Gubler Syndrome*

The Millard–Gubler syndrome is due to a lesion in the pons affecting the sixth nerve nucleus, corticospinal tract, and intra-axial portion of the seventh nerve. Clinical findings include ipsilateral lateral rectus palsy, contralateral hemiplegia, and ipsilateral facial weakness; the seventh nerve palsy is typical of lower motoneuron seventh nerve palsies.

*Foville's Syndrome*

A lesion in the pons can affect the PPRF, corticospinal tract, and intra-axial portion of the facial nerve. Patients present with an ipsilateral facial palsy, contralateral hemiparesis, and gaze palsy to the side of the lesion.

*Locked-In Syndrome*

Locked-in syndrome is most commonly due to basilar artery thrombosis, although it can also be due to pontine hemorrhage or infarction or central pontine myelinolysis.

Patients present with quadriplegia and facial weakness. Often, the only motor power is of vertical eye movements and eye closure. Patients are often misdiagnosed as being in a coma because of the absence of response to verbal command, but if the examiner is careful to test by eye blink or eye movement, the patient is found to be awake and able to take in sensory information. Patients quickly learn to communicate by a code of these minimal movements if given the opportunity.

The differential diagnosis of locked-in syndrome includes other causes of quadriparesis including Guillain–Barré syndrome and other neuropathies, botulism, myasthenia gravis, and profound metabolic derangement. The differential diagnosis also includes true coma, persistent vegetative state (see Chapter 1), and akinetic mutism (see Chapter 1).

*Pure Motor Hemiparesis*

Lacunar infarction of the ventral aspect of the pons, the basis pontis, can especially damage the corticospinal tract fibers, leaving more dorsally located cranial nuclei and nerves spared. This condition results in contralateral hemiparesis with few or no associated signs.

The pons derives arterial supply from the basilar artery, which in turn sends circumferential arteries around the pons. These arteries send penetrating branches into the pons. Occlusion of one of these penetrating vessels is thought to be responsible for brain stem lacunar syndromes. The differential diagnosis of pure motor hemiparesis due to pontine infarction is lacunar infarction of the internal capsule or infarction of the cerebral peduncle in the midbrain.

*Clumsy Hand–Dysarthria Syndrome*
Lacunar infarction of the basis pontis may involve not only the corticospinal tract, as with pure motor hemiparesis, but also the facial nerve. Patients present with dysarthria, dysphagia, clumsiness, and corticospinal tract signs. Differential diagnosis includes lesions of the internal capsule.

**Medulla**

*Anatomy*
Figure 3.5 shows a cross-section of the medulla. There are rostral–caudal differences in organization, so the figure is slightly stylized. Important landmarks includes the corticospinal tracts, olivary nucleus, medial lemniscus, medial longitudinal fasciculus, vestibular nucleus, nucleus ambiguus, hypoglossal nucleus and nerve, nucleus of the tractus solitarius, descending sympathetic tract, spinothalamic tract, and inferior cerebellar peduncle.

The blood supply to the medulla is from branches of the vertebral arteries, since the basilar artery has not formed yet at this location. The major vessels are the posterior inferior cerebellar artery (PICA) and medial branches, which join to form the anterior spinal artery.

The corticospinal tract travels in the medullary pyramids. The corticospinal tract decussates in the medulla, with the arm axons crossing slightly rostral to the crossing of the leg axons; this arrangement allows a very localized lesion to produce corticospinal dys-

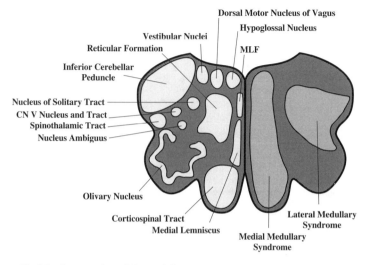

**Fig. 3.5** Cross-section of the medulla.

function affecting the ipsilateral arm and contralateral leg, although in practice, this combination is uncommon.

Underlying the olives are the olivary nuclei, which project somatosensory information to the contralateral cerebellum. Nucleus gracilis and nucleus cuneatus are in the most caudal section of the medulla, on the dorsal surface, in continuity with the dorsal columns. Outflow crosses the midline and forms the medial lemnisci. The spinothalamic tract is a continuation of the same tract in the spinal cord and stays lateral through its course in the medulla and into the pons. The nucleus ambiguus provides axons that control muscles of the pharynx and larynx via the glossopharyngeal, vagus, and accessory nerves. The solitary tract nucleus receives taste and visceral sensation input from the facial, glossopharyngeal, and vagus nerves. The descending sympathetic tract projects into the cervical cord. The MLF contains the medial vestibulospinal and reticulospinal tracts and the tectospinal tract. The restiform body forms the inferior cerebellar peduncle.

### Lesions

#### Lateral Medullary Syndrome

Lateral medullary (Wallenberg's) syndrome is usually due to occlusion of the PICA, which is a branch of the vertebral artery. Findings include ipsilateral ataxia due to damage to the inferior cerebellar peduncle and cerebellum, ipsilateral Horner's syndrome from involvement of the intrinsic sympathetic axons that descend into the cervical cord, and vertigo with nausea with or without vomiting from damage to the vestibular nuclei. Ipsilateral pharyngeal and laryngeal dysfunction produces dysarthria and dysphagia. Ipsilateral trigeminal involvement produces sensory loss on the face. Damage to the ascending spinothalamic tract produces decreased pain and temperature sensation contralateral to the lesion.

#### Medial Medullary Syndrome

The medial medullary syndrome is less common than the lateral medullary syndrome. Infarction of the medial medulla is due to occlusion of branches of the vertebral artery, which project to form the anterior spinal artery. These penetrating branches can be occluded, infarcting the pyramids, medial lemniscus, and hypoglossal nerve. Patients present with contralateral hemiparesis, contralateral loss of position and vibratory sensation, and ipsilateral paresis of the tongue.

## CEREBELLUM

### Anatomy

The cerebellum sits dorsal to the brain stem in the posterior fossa. All of its inputs and outputs pass through the brain stem. The cerebellum can be divided into several phylogenetic and physiologic divisions, but in clinical practice, the most important distinction is between disorders affecting the vermis and those affecting the cerebellar hemispheres.

The cerebellum can be divided into the anterior lobe, posterior lobe, and flocculonodular lobe. The anterior lobe is the section rostral to the primary fissure of the cerebellum. This lobe receives prominent input from the spinocerebellar pathways and is involved in gait and truncal coordination. The posterior lobe receives extensive input from the cerebral hemispheres and is concerned with coordination of individual limb movements. The flocculonodular lobe receives input from the vestibular nuclei and is concerned with proximal coordination.

Inputs to the cerebellum are largely through the middle and inferior cerebellar peduncles, although the ventral spinocerebellar tract and a few other minor afferent tracts pass through the superior cerebellar peduncle. Outflow from the cerebellum is through the superior cerebellar peduncle. Axons from the cerebellar cortex project to the deep nuclei, which in turn project axons through the superior cerebellar peduncle to the contralateral red nucleus, contralateral ventrolateral nucleus of the thalamus, reticular formation, and vestibular nuclei.

The cerebellum is involved in control of movement; the flocculonodular lobe, anterior lobe, and especially the vermis are involved in control of gait and truncal movement (Figure 3.6). The posterior lobe, especially the hemispheres, is involved in coordinating movements of individual ipsilateral limbs.

### Lesions

The first important distinction in clinical practice is among lesions that mostly affect the vermis, that mostly affect the cerebellar hemispheres, or that diffusely affect the cerebellum. The second important distinction is between lesions that affect only the cerebellum and lesions that affect the brain stem and/or other neural structures.

Diagnosis of cerebellar dysfunction depends on history and examination, as with any neurological structure. Acute onset of

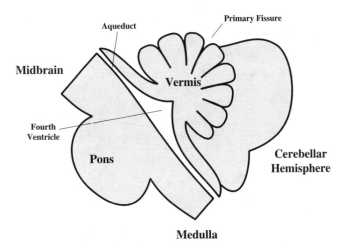

**Fig. 3.6** The relationship of the vermis and cerebellar hemisphere to the brain stem is shown.

cerebellar ataxia suggests a vascular insult, whether infarction or hemorrhage. Slowly progressive ataxia has a wide differential diagnosis, although the most important causes are alcoholic cerebellar degeneration, tumors, and hereditary cerebellar degeneration.

Lesion of the vermis produces gait ataxia characterized by a broad-based stance and impaired placing of the limbs when walking. Compensatory movements can produce a truncal tremor with stance and gait. Movements of the individual limbs show good coordination. Nystagmus is sometimes seen.

Lesion of the cerebellar hemisphere produces limb ataxia ipsilateral to the lesion. Movements are jerky and often fragmented. Gait is broad-based, and the patient tends to fall to the side of the lesion.

Repetitive movements are irregular, lacking the rhythm and consistency of normal movements. Tremor of the ipsilateral limbs that is prominent with movement can develop, as seen on finger–nose–finger testing.

### Cerebellar Stroke

Cerebellar stroke presents with acute onset of cerebellar ataxia, often associated with vertigo, nystagmus, and other signs referable to brain stem dysfunction. Infarction can directly involve the brain stem in addition to the cerebellum; hemorrhage can result in brain stem compression and is a neurosurgical emergency. Clinical differentiation of hemorrhage from infarction of the cerebellum is imperfect; presumption of infarction may delay the surgery necessary for cerebellar hemorrhage, so early imaging is necessary in patients with cerebellar stroke.

#### Infarction Producing Cerebellar Ataxia

The cerebellum receives its blood supply via the superior cerebellar artery, AICA, and PICA. These three vessels anastomose extensively on the surface of the cerebellum.

PICA infarction is discussed earlier in this chapter. AICA infarction produces ipsilateral ataxia from damage to the cerebellar hemisphere and peduncle, along with brain stem findings such as vertigo, nystagmus, and ipsilateral Horner's syndrome. Patients may have ipsilateral facial weakness from CN VII involvement, along with deafness and facial sensory loss due to trigeminal nucleus and tract involvement, with loss of the corneal reflex. Superior cerebellar artery infarction produces ipsilateral ataxia plus nystagmus, vertigo, Horner's syndrome, and intention tremor and may produce contralateral hearing loss due to involvement of the crossed lateral lemniscus.

Cerebellar ataxia develops as a result of many brain stem stroke syndromes; in some, the cerebellum is directly infarcted while in others the ataxia is due to damage to cerebellar inflow or outflow tracts. For example, midbrain infarction with damage to the red nucleus can produce contralateral cerebellar ataxia, and lateral medullary infarction with damage to the inferior cerebellar peduncle causes ipsilateral cerebellar ataxia. In patients with the acute-onset cerebellar ataxia thought to be secondary to stroke, associated brain stem signs must be sought; these signs will aid in localizing the area of damage.

*Cerebellar Hemorrhage*

Cerebellar hemorrhage may present with cerebellar ataxia but many patients have signs referable to mass effect, which produces brain stem compression. Common symptoms include occipital headache, vertigo, gait and/or limb ataxia, nausea with or without vomiting, and diplopia. Signs include nystagmus, gaze palsies, skew deviation, ataxia, hyperreflexia with upward plantar responses, facial weakness, and decreased level of consciousness.

### Alcoholic Cerebellar Degeneration

Alcoholics may develop gait ataxia due to degeneration of the rostral vermis. This degeneration has a characteristic appearance at autopsy, which may be seen even on MRI sagittal images of the vermis; atrophy of the rostral segments is far out of proportion to atrophy of the remainder of the vermis.

Patients present with gait ataxia with little or no arm ataxia. Leg coordination is impaired on heel–knee–shin testing.

### Tumors

Tumors may affect the midline or hemispheres of the cerebellum. Tumors of the midline will mainly affect gait, while tumors of the hemispheres will produce limb ataxia. The mass effect of all cerebellar tumors can result in global cerebellar dysfunction and ultimately distortion of the brain stem with resultant brain stem signs. Obstructive hydrocephalus can develop with deformation and eventual obliteration of the fourth ventricle.

Cerebellar tumors in children are usually primary and include cystic astrocytomas in the hemispheres, ependymoma, primitive neuroectodermal tumors invading the midline of the cerebellum, and medulloblastoma. Cerebellar tumors in adults are more frequently metastatic and may be midline or lateral. Meningiomas can produce cerebellar appendicular or gait ataxia, depending on location; a large proportion of meningiomas are incidental findings on imaging studies in patients being imaged for other reasons. Oligodendrogliomas are rare in the posterior fossa.

### Cerebellar Degenerations

Cerebellar degenerations are not common and they are frequently not recognized; many patients are misdiagnosed as having Parkinson's disease or stroke. The degeneration may be hereditary, paraneoplastic, or of unknown etiology.

Patients present with gradually progressive ataxia that affects gait and limb movements, indicating diffuse cerebellar involvement. Cerebellar degenerations are suggested by prominent cerebellar ataxia with other neurologic deficits being less impressive. Important cerebellar degenerations are discussed below; in these degenerations, the cerebellar signs are only a portion of the neurologic findings.

#### Early-Onset Inherited Ataxias
FRIEDREICH'S ATAXIA

Friedreich's ataxia is an autosomal recessive disorder characterized by cerebellar degeneration and other neurologic findings, including peripheral neuropathy, corticospinal tract signs, and cardiomyopathy. Patients have an increased incidence of optic atrophy, diabetes mellitus, and sensorineural deafness. Onset is usually between 8 and 15 years of age.

Patients present with cerebellar symptoms and signs; on examination, associated findings are detected. Family history must be taken in these patients, as in all patients with progressive cerebellar ataxia.

Diagnosis is by clinical findings. Patients with Charcot–Marie–Tooth disease or hereditary motor–sensory neuropathy I may be misdiagnosed as having Friedreich's ataxia, since they may appear ataxic because of their severe neuropathy.

RAMSAY HUNT SYNDROME

Ramsay Hunt syndrome usually has autosomal recessive inheritance, although occasional families have autosomal dominant inheritance. Patients present with cerebellar ataxia plus myoclonus.

OTHER EARLY-ONSET INHERITED ATAXIAS

The other early-onset inherited disorders are much less common than Friedreich's ataxia. Patients present with cerebellar ataxia, but they do not have the other physical findings of Freidreich's ataxia, such as peripheral neuropathy.

*Late-Onset Inherited Ataxias*

This group of disorders encompasses many clinical presentations. Patients have other neurologic findings in addition to cerebellar ataxia in almost all cases.

AUTOSOMAL DOMINANT CEREBELLAR ATAXIAS

Autosomal dominant cerebellar ataxia (ADCA) comprises three syndromes differentiated by associated neurologic signs. ADCA I presents with relatively pure cerebellar ataxia, but later dementia or supranuclear ophthalmoplegia may be seen. Onset is usually in the third or fourth decade.

ADCA II is associated with pigmentary retinal degeneration. ADCA III is not associated with ophthalmoplegia or dementia and has an onset later then ADCA I, in the sixth decade or later.

*Idiopathic Progressive Ataxias*

Sporadic cases of progressive cerebellar ataxia with other neurologic signs have as previously been classified as olivopontocerebellar atrophy (OPCA); however, the term "olivopontocerebellar atrophy" has been rejected by some because it does not completely describe the degeneration seen. Cerebellar ataxia has its onset in middle or old age. Associated signs may include dementia, peripheral neuropathy, supranuclear ophthalmoplegia, and parkinsonism

The diagnosis is suspected when a patient presents with cerebellar ataxia plus signs that cannot be explained by abnormalities in the cerebellum or pons, such as parkinsonism or peripheral neuropathy. Imaging studies are almost always indicated to rule out a posterior fossa mass or infiltrating lesion. EMG may document the neuropathy.

*Paraneoplastic Cerebellar Degeneration*
Cerebellar ataxia occurs in children with neuroblastoma as a remote effect of tumor. Patients present with gait and limb ataxia plus opsoclonus.

Cerebellar ataxia occurs in adults with cancers of the lung, breast, and/or gastrointestinal tract and with lymphoma. Patients present with gait and limb ataxia with nystagmus. Degeneration of Purkinje cells of the cerebellum is found at autopsy.

Diagnosis is made clinically after imaging studies fail to show tumor in the posterior fossa. Circulating antibodies can be measured.

### *Peri-Infectious Cerebellar Dysfunction*

Acute cerebellar ataxia can develop after viral infection, especially varicella. Patients present with cerebellar ataxia affecting appendicular and gait function, nystagmus, and occasionally opsoclonus and head tremor. Except for the cerebellar signs, the neurologic examination is usually normal. It is unclear whether this ataxia is mediated directly by the virus or by an immune-mediated attack.

## CRANIAL NERVE, BRAIN STEM, AND CEREBELLAR SYNDROMES

### Arnold–Chiari Malformation

The Arnold–Chiari malformation is a disorder of early development of the craniocervical junction in which the cerebellar tonsils extend through the foramen magnum. In many patients, this malformation is an incidental finding on MRI, but it can become symptomatic through compression of the cervicomedullary junction or hydrocephalus. Arnold–Chiari malformation is divided into the following types:

- Type I: herniation of the cerebellar tonsils with no other neurologic involvement

- Type II: herniation of the cerebellar tonsils along with caudal displacement of the medulla
- Type III: cervical spina bifida with a cerebellar encephalocele

Type III is usually obvious at birth. Diagnosis of types I and II is less obvious and should be considered in patients with symptoms of hydrocephalus and/or cervicomedullary junction lesion, including headache with nausea with or without vomiting, ataxia, head tilt, pain in the neck and shoulders, and dysfunction of the lower cranial nerves. Corticospinal tract signs may be present. Nystagmus is common with medullary compression.

## Dandy–Walker Syndrome

Dandy–Walker syndrome is agenesis of the cerebellar vermis with a cystic region in the dorsal aspect of the posterior fossa that communicates with the fourth ventricle. Hydrocephalus develops in childhood or in adult life.

Patients present in childhood with large heads. Associated neurologic findings include ataxia, corticospinal tract signs, nystagmus, and cranial nerve palsies. If the hydrocephalus develops in adult life, patients present with typical signs of hydrocephalus. The majority of patients have other neurologic developmental disorders, including agenesis of the corpus callosum, hererotopias, aqueductal stenosis, and pachygyria of the cerebral cortex (see Chapter 1).

## Foster Kennedy Syndrome

The Foster Kennedy syndrome is usually due to a tumor affecting the inferior frontal region, including meningiomas of the olfactory groove or sphenoid ridge. The clinical triad consists of the following:

- Ipsilateral anosmia
- Ipsilateral optic atrophy
- Contralateral papilledema

Anosmia is due to involvement of the olfactory bulb or tract. Optic atrophy is from chronic compression of the ipsilateral optic nerve. Contralateral papilledema is from pressure on the other optic nerve, which is less affected than the ipsilateral nerve because of distance from the origin of the lesion.

## Cavernous Sinus Syndrome

The cavernous sinus contains the internal carotid artery, the venous sinus itself, and cranial nerves III, IV, V, and VI. All of these can be affected by a lesion in the cavernous sinus. Of the divisions of CN V, V1 (ophthalmic division of trigeminal) is most likely to be involved, while V3 (mandibular division of trigeminal) is least likely to be involved because of its short course in the sinus before exiting.

Cavernous sinus lesions may present as painful or painless ophthalmoplegia. Occasionally, the pain may precede the ophthalmoparesis.

## Tolosa–Hunt Syndrome

Tolosa–Hunt syndrome is due to a lesion in the region of the cavernous sinus. Patients present with retro-orbital pain and have a combination of palsies of the trochlear nerve, the abducens nerve, and the ophthalmic and maxillary divisions of the trigeminal nerve. The differential diagnosis includes other cavernous sinus lesions, pituitary tumors, and pituitary apoplexy (Figure 3.7).

## Superior Orbital Fissure Syndrome

Superior orbital fissure syndrome resembles cavernous sinus in that all three ocular motor nerves may be affected. However, proptosis is common.

## Cerebellopontine Angle Syndrome

Lesions at the cerebellopontine angle may include acoustic neuromas, meningiomas, vascular malformations, neuromas of the trigeminal, facial, or glossopharyngeal nerves, intrinsic tumors of the brain stem such as gliomas, and chronic meningeal involvement of tumor or an infectious agent.

Symptoms depend on the structures involved, but common symptoms include ipsilateral facial numbness from trigeminal involvement, ipsilateral hemiataxia from involvement of the cerebel-

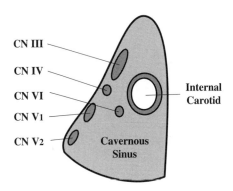

**Fig. 3.7** Coronal section of the cavernous sinus shows the anatomical relationship between cranial nerves III, IV, V, and VI and the internal carotid artery.

lum or cerebellar peduncle, tinnitus, and hearing loss. Tinnitus is a common presenting complaint, while hearing loss is often only found on examination. Facial nerve involvement can occur but is uncommon, especially early in the course. Compression or infiltration of the brain stem can produce contralateral weakness with corticospinal tract signs.

### Gradenigo's Syndrome

Gradenigo's syndrome is dysfunction of CN V1 and the sixth nerve, usually due to involvement where the two nerves are near one another in the temporal bone. Patients have pain in a V1 distribution associated with lateral rectus palsy.

### Basilar Thrombosis

Thrombosis of the basilar artery results in extensive infarction of the pons and midbrain and is usually fatal. Patients present with coma, quadriplegia, and horizontal gaze palsies. Some patients with less extensive damage may present with the locked-in syndrome. Basilar thrombosis is suspected by the bilateral brain stem signs, with localization at and above the level of the pons.

## Olivopontocerebellar Atrophy and Multiple System Atrophy

OPCA is characterized by ataxia and spasticity associated with other neurologic findings, including central ocular motor palsies, myoclonus, other cranial nerve palsies, dyskinesias, and visual loss from retinal degeneration. Not all findings are present in all patients. Degeneration is prominent in the medullary olives, pons, and cerebellar cortex. As already discussed, the term "olivopontocerebellar atrophy" is not used by some clinicians because it insufficiently describes the signs and pathology. OPCA is classified with the inherited cerebellar ataxias (see above).

"Multiple system atrophy" is sometimes used to describe a specific diagnostic entity, although this use is controversial. The syndrome consists of autonomic failure, parkinsonism, cerebellar ataxia, and corticospinal tract signs. Neural degeneration is widespread. Multiple system atrophy is probably best thought of as one of the "parkinsonism plus" syndromes, along with OPCA, Shy–Drager syndrome (discussed below), and progressive supranuclear palsy (see Chapter 1).

## Shy–Drager Syndrome

Shy–Drager syndrome presents with orthostatic hypotension plus neurologic symptoms that may include parkinsonism, axonal neuropathy, cerebellar ataxia, and/or spasticity. Preganglionic autonomic neurons in the intermediolateral cell column are degenerated, resulting in prominent autonomic dysfunction. Impotence and urinary and gastrointestinal dysfunction are typical.

Suspicion is key to the diagnosis. Shy–Drager syndrome should be thought of in patients showing parkinsonism along with signs of neuropathy, especially in the presence of severe orthostatic hypotension. Orthostatic hypotension may develop in Parkinson's disease but not to the severity typical of Shy–Drager syndrome.

## Top-of-the-Basilar Syndrome

Top-of-the-basilar syndrome is due to occlusion of the distal basilar artery as it bifurcates into the left and right posterior cerebral arteries. The occlusion is usually due to an embolus ascending in the vertebral arteries to the basilar arteries. Symptoms and signs are mainly due to infarction of the occipital lobes and midbrain, thalamus, and medial aspect of the temporal lobe. Findings include cortical blindness from bilateral occipital lobe damage, pupil and eye movement defects from midbrain damage, and memory dysfunction from temporal lobe damage. Damage to descending corticospinal tracts can produce corticospinal tract signs. Sensory findings can be due to damage to ascending tracts as well as thalamic damage.

Eye movement abnormalities include paralysis of vertical gaze, convergence, and skew deviation. Pupillary abnormalities include irregular or asymmetric pupils, often with decreased responsiveness. If the occipital lobe involvement is incomplete, patients may have hemianopia or other incomplete visual field defects.

# 4

# Spinal Cord

## ANATOMY

The spinal cord serves as a conduit for information relayed between the brain stem and peripheral nervous system. In addition to this purely conductive function, there is substantial neural processing at segmental levels of the spinal cord.

### Segmental Anatomy

Figure 4.1 shows a spinal cord segment in cross-section. The clinically most important aspects of segmental anatomy are the following:

- The centrally located gray matter, which consists of motoneurons for the muscles innervated by that segment of cord plus interneurons that control segmental reflexes and modulate ascending and descending information
- The peripherally located white matter, which consists of tracts of axons that ascend and descend in the spinal cord
- The dorsal gray matter, which is involved in processing input to the cord, while the ventral gray matter contains the lower motoneurons

### Tracts

There is a multiplicity of tracts ascending and descending the spinal cord, as shown in Figure 4.1 and detailed in Table 4.1. Only the most important tracts are discussed here:

- Corticospinal tract
- Bulbospinal tracts (including rubrospinal, reticulospinal, tectospinal, and vestibulospinal tracts)
- Anterolateral tracts

- Dorsal columns
- Spinocerebellar tracts

The clinically most important aspects of tract anatomy are as follows:

- The corticospinal tract is mostly already crossed, so the descending axons project to ipsilateral motoneurons.
- The dorsal columns convey large-fiber sensations of vibration and proprioception and ascend uncrossed.
- The anterolateral tract conveys pain and temperature sensation and crosses before ascending.

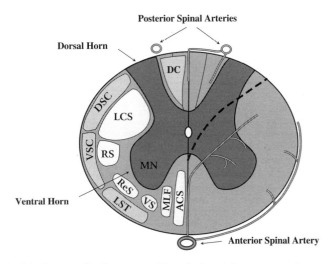

**Fig. 4.1** Cross-sectional anatomy of the spinal cord shows some major tracts on the left side of the figure. The lateral corticospinal (LCS), anterior corticospinal (ACS), rubrospinal (RS), reticulospinal (ReS), medial longitudinal fasciculus (MLF), and vestibulospinal (VS) are descending tracts. The dorsal columns (DC), lateral spinothalamic (LST), dorsal spinocerebellar (DSC), and ventral spinocerebellar (VSC) are ascending tracts. The motoneurons (MN) are in the anterior horns.

**Table 4.1 Spinal Tracts**

| Tract | Function | Results of Lesion |
|-------|----------|-------------------|
| Anterolateral tract | Pain and temperature sensation; poorly localized touch sensation | Loss of pain and temperature sensation; preserved touch, though it may have a different quality |
| Bulbospinal tract | Postural stability and co-activation of axial and appendicular muscles | Isolated lesions uncommon |
| Corticospinal tract | Initiation and maintenance of movement; especially important for fine, precise movement | Weakness, spasticity, upward plantar responses |
| Dorsal columns | Vibration and proprioceptive sensation; localized touch sensation | Loss of vibration and proprioceptive sensation |
| Spinocerebellar tract | Proprioceptive and touch sensation; perception of body in physical space | Ataxia with fragmented appendicular movements; isolated lesions uncommon |

### Corticospinal Tract

The cell bodies of the corticospinal tract are in the cerebral cortex; about one third of them are from the precentral gyrus (area 4), one third are from area 6, anterior to area 4, and one third are from areas 1, 2, and 3, posterior to the central sulcus. The cell bodies descend through the cerebral peduncle and brain stem, and three quarters of them decussate in the medulla. The crossed axons descend in the lateral corticospinal tract in the lateral funiculus of the spinal cord. At various levels, axons leave the tract and terminate in the spinal gray matter on motoneurons and interneurons of the spinal cord.

Corticospinal axons that do not decussate in the medulla descend in the anterior corticospinal tract in the medial aspect of the ventral funiculus. Axons leave the tract at various spinal levels, some crossing through the ventral commissure and others remaining uncrossed, to terminate in the anterior horns.

The crossed lateral corticospinal tract projects to neurons that control appendicular muscles. The anterior corticospinal tract, with crossed and uncrossed fibers, projects to motoneurons controlling axial muscles. In theory, activation of a cortical region results in movement of a contralateral limb along with stabilization of the body through activation of bilateral axial muscles. Limb movement is primarily controlled by the lateral corticospinal tract, and axial stabilization is accomplished by the anterior corticospinal tract with bilateral projections.

### Bulbospinal Tracts

While the corticospinal tract is seen as the main motor outflow of the brain, other pathways are of great importance. Pathways from the cortex project not only to spinal neurons, but also to bulbar centers, which in turn project to spinal interneurons. Brain stem centers also receive sensory input to aid in feedback control of movement; accurate movements cannot be made without sensory feedback.

Descending pathways from the brain stem are divided into medial and lateral divisions. The medial pathway consists of the reticulospinal, vestibulospinal, and tectospinal tracts, which descend in the ventral funiculus. The medial pathways mostly activate proximal muscles, especially antigravity muscles. The reticulospinal pathways are probably involved in postural control of axial muscles during movement. The vestibulospinal pathways are also involved in maintenance of posture. The tectospinal pathway is involved in integration of head and eye movement with body movement.

The lateral brain stem descending pathway consists mainly of the rubrospinal tract, which originates in the red nucleus and then crosses and descends in the lateral funiculus. Lateral pathways innervate mainly distal muscles. The rubrospinal tract is involved in control of fine movements, but much of this function is assumed by corticospinal projections in humans; the rubrospinal tract has greater importance for fine movements in lower primates.

### Anterolateral Tracts

Afferents conveying mainly pain and temperature terminate in the dorsal horn, where they synapse on second-order neurons that cross and ascend in the contralateral anterolateral tracts. The anterolateral tracts consist of the anterior spinothalamic tract and lateral spinothalamic tract. Many of the axons terminate in the thalamus (spinothalamic tract), but some terminate in the reticular formation of the pons and medulla (spinoreticular tract) and in the midbrain (spinomesencephalic tract). Some tactile sensation is carried by the anterolateral system, but it is more poorly localized than that carried in the dorsal columns.

### Dorsal Columns

The dorsal columns form the dorsal funiculus. They are composed of central axons of primary afferent neurons with cell bodies in the dorsal root ganglia, with a small contribution of ascending neurons with cell bodies in the dorsal horn. These neurons carry tactile sensation, including the large-fiber sensations of vibration and proprioception, in addition to touch. The dorsal columns are topographically organized with the legs being represented medially and the arms proximally in upper cord regions.

The dorsal columns terminate in the dorsal column nuclei. Axons from the leg terminate in the nucleus gracilis and axons from the arm terminate in the nucleus cuneatus, where they synapse on neurons whose axons cross and form the medial lemniscus, which projects to the thalamus.

### Spinocerebellar Tracts

The spinocerebellar tracts are involved in control of movement of the body in physical space and movement of body parts in relation to each other. Spinal afferents carrying proprioceptive and touch information enter the dorsal horn and synapse in the dorsal horn, and the second-order neurons ascend in the spinocerebellar tracts, which are located in the most lateral aspect of the spinal cord. The ascending fibers from the dorsal spinocerebellar tract enter the brain stem, then enter the cerebellum via the inferior cerebellar peduncle. The axons of the ventral spinocerebellar tract ascend higher in the brain stem, then turn to descend into the cerebellum via the superior cerebellar peduncle.

## Vascular Anatomy of the Spinal Cord

The arterial supply to the spinal cord is from multiple levels, beginning with branches of the vertebral arteries that fuse to form the anterospinal artery, which runs along the anterior or ventral side of the cord. This artery receives additional vascular supply from segmental vessels. A major vessel is the artery of Adamkiewicz, which arises from the aorta and usually enters between T9 and L2 and supplies the anterior spinal artery.

The anterior spinal artery supplies the anterior two thirds of the spinal cord, including most of the gray matter, descending tracts, both lateral and anterior spinothalamic tracts, and the spinocerebellar tracts. The posterior spinal arteries lie on the posterior or dorsal surface of the spinal cord but are not as continuous as the anterior cerebral artery. Looking at the dorsal surface of the cord, the posterior spinal arteries appear to be major components of a network of vessels with interconnections. These vessels supply the dorsal columns and part of the dorsal horns.

The venous drainage of the spinal cord is of less clinical importance than the arterial supply. The venous plexus drains through radicular veins.

## LESIONS

### Guide to Localization

A lesion of the spinal cord is suspected in the presence of one or more of the following (Table 4.2):

- Bilateral leg motor and/or sensory loss without arm involvement; differential diagnosis includes a parasagittal cerebral lesion.

**Table 4.2 Spinal Lesions**

| Lesion | Symptoms |
| --- | --- |
| Anterior spinal artery syndrome | Paralysis and loss of pain and temperature sensation below the lesion; preservation of vibration and proprioception; level is usually between T9 and L1 |
| Brown–Séquard (spinal hemisection) syndrome | *Ipsilateral:* segmental lower motoneuron dysfunction, loss of vibration and proprioception below lesion; corticospinal tract signs below level of the lesion; *Contralateral:* loss of pain and temperature sensation |
| Cauda equina syndrome | Asymmetric pain and sensory loss affecting caudal nerve roots, especially L4–S2; bowel and bladder changes with severe disease |
| Central cord syndrome (usually cervical spine) | Weakness of arms with relative preservation of legs; corticospinal tract signs in legs but not arms; frequently painful in arms |
| Neoplastic cord compression | Pain in spine region; ultimately, weakness and sensory loss below level of lesion |
| Neoplastic meningitis | Multifocal motor and sensory loss in distribution of individual dermatomes; pain common with nerve root infiltration |
| Spinal stenosis | Back pain, often exacerbated by walking; patchy weakness and reflex changes in the legs, usually in a dermatomal distribution |
| Syrinx | Loss of pain and temperature sensation at level of the lesion, followed by lower motoneuron signs, then long track signs and more definite myelopathy |

- Dissociated motor and sensory finding—that is, upper motoneuron signs on one side and pain and temperature loss on the other side
- Back pain and neurologic deficit below the level of the pain
- New onset of back pain in a patient with a known malignancy

All of the following syndromes are most commonly caused by a lesion affecting the spinal cord. The differential diagnosis is usually large, but these are the most common causes of cord lesions:

- Herniated disk
- Spondylosis with resultant spinal stenosis
- Trauma
- Tumor
- Transverse myelitis
- Multiple sclerosis

Localizing the lesion to the portion of the cord affected aids in diagnosis. The differential diagnosis is narrowed by deciding exactly how the cord is affected through the following signs:

- Corticospinal tract signs
- Segmental gray matter signs
- Nerve root involvement

Corticospinal tract signs, including weakness, spasticity, and a sensory level below the level of the lesion indicate dysfunction of the white matter tracts. This combination predominates in demyelinating diseases, such as transverse myelitis and multiple sclerosis, and it can be an early sign of any cause of extrinsic cord compression.

Atrophy of muscles innervated by one segmental level usually is due to nerve root involvement, but if the denervation spans two or three levels and is bilateral, then a midline gray matter lesion is suspected. Gray matter lesions include syrinx and intraparenchymal tumors.

The motor and sensory levels of the deficit are usually fairly accurate in localizing the rostral–caudal extent of the lesion; however, a lesion may be significantly above the level of the deficit. For example, leg weakness with a sensory level in the midthoracic region may be due to a lesion low in the cervical cord; imaging only of the thoracic region will miss the lesion. Figure 4.2 shows the regions of the spinal cord affected by some important disorders.

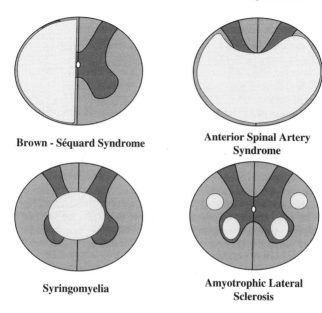

**Fig. 4.2** Cross-sections of the spinal cord show areas affected by some important disorders.

## Tumors Affecting the Spinal Cord

Tumors affecting the spinal cord can be classified into the following categories:

- Extradural
- Intradural but extramedullary
- Intramedullary

Extradural tumors are the most common, and they are usually due to metastases from systemic neoplasms. Lung, breast, renal, and gastrointestinal tumors first metastasize to the bone and subsequently expand into the spinal canal, producing extrinsic cord compression. Involvement of a local nerve root may result in radicular pain, weakness, and sensory loss. The vast majority of tumors affecting the spine have associated back pain, so absence of back pain would be strong, though not absolute, evidence against a spinal tumor. Lymphomas extend from the paravertebral region through a nerve root foramen into the spinal canal, also producing cord compression. Radicular symptoms are expected.

Intradural but extramedullary tumors are usually neurofibromas or meningiomas. They produce all of the signs and symptoms of extrinsic cord compression, although there may be signs of nerve root compression as well.

Intramedullary tumors are usually gliomas. They frequently produce initial symptoms by involvement of the gray matter. With progression, there is involvement of the white matter with subsequent development of corticospinal tract signs. Back pain may be present, but it is less common than with extradural tumors. Radicular pain is unusual with intramedullary tumors.

Diagnosis of spinal tumors is usually by magnetic resonance imaging (MRI); however, if the expected lesion is not found, complete myelography may be indicated.

### Brown–Séquard Syndrome

Spinal cord hemisection is known as Brown–Séquard syndrome. The classic description is based on complete surgical section of one lateral half of the cord, and it is a lesion rarely seen in clinical practice. However, elements of the Brown–Séquard syndrome are seen in some patients with traumatic injuries, tumors, asymmetric spondylosis, and, rarely, infections of the spine.

Ipsilateral findings at the level of the lesion include weakness of muscles innervated by this dermatome. Below the level of the lesion, deficits of vibration and proprioception, muscle weakness, and corticospinal tract signs are seen. There are no contralateral findings at the level of the lesion; however, below the level of the lesion, there are deficits in pain and temperature sensations.

The most important clinical findings for diagnosis of the syndrome are those below the level of the lesion. Deficit and pain help localize the dermatomal level of the lesion.

### Tabes Dorsalis and Syphilitic Myelitis

Tabes dorsalis is due to involvement of the dorsal roots by late neurosyphilis. There is meningeal inflammation along with inflammatory changes in the dorsal roots. Damage to these axons results in atrophy of the dorsal root ganglia and dorsal columns. Patients present with sensory ataxia; that is, their balance and gait difficulties are due to lack of correct sensory information regarding limb position. Classically there is a slapping gait. Reflexes are depressed, as is common with sensory deficits.

Involvement of the ventral roots may produce weakness and atrophy, but these findings are much less prominent than the sensory findings. Associated neurologic findings are clues to the diagnosis. The Argyll Robertson pupil is discussed in Chapter 3, and other pupillary abnormalities can be seen as well. Charcot joints are joints that have been destroyed due to absence of detection of pain. Other cranial neuropathies may be present, producing ptosis, facial weakness, and/or hearing loss. Bowel and bladder reflexes are impaired because of damage to afferents. However, there are no findings to suggest corticospinal damage.

A more rare cause of spinal cord dysfunction is syphilitic myelitis, which presents as progressive weakness and spasticity below the level of involvement. This condition tends to occur earlier in the course of syphilis than tabes dorsalis.

### Transverse Myelitis

Transverse myelitis is a clinical syndrome that may include several disorders. Patients present with an onset of myelopathy that progresses over hours to days. Back pain and vague sensory symptoms may precede objective signs of myelopathy. A minority of patients will report a preceding febrile illness, but this is not a useful clinical feature.

Transverse myelitis is an isolated entity in most patients. Only some seven percent subsequently develop multiple sclerosis.

## Multiple Sclerosis

Multiple sclerosis (MS) is characterized by zones of demyelination with preservation of axons. The spinal cord is often though not invariably involved, producing myelopathy that resembles transverse myelitis. The diagnosis is suspected by evidence of history or examination of other demyelinating lesions either in the past or subsequent to the myelopathy. Common associated symptoms include visual loss, hemiparesis or hemisensory loss, and ataxia.

Diagnosis of MS is established by clinical criteria, and the role of imaging, though it has been intensively studied, is still controversial. When a patient presents with myelopathy, MRI of the head is often ordered, but the diagnosis of MS should not be made even if areas of increased signal intensity on T2-weighted images are seen.

## Syringomyelia

Syringomyelia is a cyst in the spinal gray matter that extends longitudinally over several segments. It is different from hydromyelia, which is abnormal enlargement of the central canal. Syrinx is most commonly due to a Arnold–Chiari malformation, which is thought to produce the cyst by causing blockage of cerebrospinal fluid flow, pressure waves within the central canal, subsequent rupture of the central canal into the surrounding parenchyma, and ultimate formation of the cyst. The mass effect of the syrinx will initially damage the crossing fibers destined for the anterior spinothalamic tract, which convey pain and temperature sensation. Subsequently, damage to the gray matter at the levels of the syrinx will produce motoneuron degeneration. With more severe enlargement, compression of white matter tracts will produce signs below the level of the lesion, including spasticity and sensory loss.

Patients present with loss of pain and temperature sensation at the levels of the lesion; with cervical syrinx, this loss occurs across the shoulders and arms, sometimes described as a cape or shawl distribution. Weakness from lower motoneuron degeneration at the level of the lesion develops. With white matter compression, spasticity below the lesion and sensory loss below the lesion develops; at this stage, it is difficult to differentiate a syrinx on clinical grounds from other causes of myelopathy.

Differential diagnosis includes other causes of myelopathy including tumors. Intraparenchymal tumors, usually gliomas, may present in a fashion indistinguishable from syrinx. Diagnosis is by MRI.

**Anterior Horn Cell Disease**

Motoneurons are also called "anterior horn cells" even though there are other types of neurons in the anterior horn of the spinal cord. The three most important motoneuron diseases are poliomyelitis, spinal muscular atrophy (SMA) and amyotrophic lateral sclerosis (ALS).

*Poliomyelitis*

Polio is due to infection of the spinal cord and brain stem by an enterovirus. Polio is unfortunately still occasionally seen in nonimmunized patients. In immunized patients, polio is due to either incomplete inactivation of the virus contained in the vaccine or a type of virus not included in the vaccine.

The virus infects motoneurons of the spinal cord and/or brain stem, producing weakness and atrophy of affected muscles. The weakness is commonly asymmetric, with preferential involvement of distal muscles. Reflexes are depressed, usually absent, differentiating this finding from the results of a central lesion.

Bulbar involvement occurs in about 15 percent of patients with polio. Cranial nerves prominently affected are the facial, glossopharyngeal, and vagus. Involvement of the reticular formation produces impaired respiration. Patients may develop encephalitic polio, presenting with impaired level of consciousness, but this is a rare occurrence.

*Spinal Muscular Atrophy*

SMA usually presents in young life, from the neonatal period to young adulthood; age of onset probably reflects rate of progression of the motoneuron degeneration rather than different pathophysiological entities. Nevertheless, SMA is considered to be three entities: infantile-onset SMA (Werdnig–Hoffman disease), juvenile-onset SMA (Kugelberg–Welander disease) and adult-onset SMA. All three are characterized by progressive degeneration of motoneurons.

Adults and older children present with progressive proximal weakness and muscle atrophy, especially in the legs. Infants present with hypotonia and weakness of facial and pharyngeal muscles. Tendon reflexes are reduced because of the decreased number of functioning motor units. Sensory function is normal.

SMA is most commonly inherited through autosomal recessive inheritance, although some patients with adult onset and rare patients with juvenile onset have autosomal dominant inheritance.

Differential diagnosis of SMA includes many myopathies and neuropathies. The purely motor character of the findings eliminates most neuropathies. Proximal predominance is common in SMA, so this cannot be used to differentiate it from myopathies. Electromyography shows different patterns in myopathy and motoneuron degeneration and therefore can confirm clinical differentiation between motoneuron diseases, such as SMA, and myopathy.

Differentiation of SMA from ALS is by absence of corticospinal tract signs. Differentiation of adult-onset SMA from progressive muscular atrophy (PMA) is difficult, but the latter usually presents with very asymmetric weakness, which often involves only one limb for years. Bulbar involvement with PMA is unusual.

### *Amyotrophic Lateral Sclerosis*

ALS is characterized by degeneration of spinal and bulbar motoneurons, plus degeneration of upper motoneurons. As a result, patients have weakness, atrophy, and fasciculations characteristic of lower motoneuron disease plus upper motoneuron signs, including hyperreflexia and upward plantar responses. Differential diagnosis includes SMA; ALS is differentiated from SMA by the presence of corticospinal tract signs in ALS. Differentiation from cervical spondylosis is discussed below.

### *Progressive Muscular Atrophy*

PMA is thought to be a variant of ALS, and it accounts for approximately 10 percent of patients with ALS. Patients present with atrophy and weakness of limb muscles. Later in the course, generalized muscular atrophy and fasciculations develop.

## Vascular Disease

Vascular disease of the spinal cord is uncommon; when present, it can be difficult to diagnose clinically. History is as important as physical examination. The abrupt onset of a deficit localized to the spinal cord in the absence of trauma suggests a vascular event. The most important spinal vascular syndromes are infarction due to occlusion of the anterior spinal artery and hemorrhage from vascular malformations and trauma.

### *Infarction*

#### *Anterior Spinal Artery Syndrome*

Probably the most common spinal vascular syndrome is infarction due to compression of the vessels by mass lesions, which is the reason mass lesions may produce acute onset or worsening of symptoms. Occlusion of the anterior spinal artery produces infarction of most of the spinal cord, excluding the dorsal aspect of the dorsal horn and dorsal columns. The occlusion is commonly due to damage to the artery of Adamkiewicz; the artery can be occluded as it arises from the aorta. Cross-clamping of the aorta is a common cause of infarction.

Patients present with paralysis below the level of the lesion. Sensory findings are important and include deficit in pain and temperature sensation below the level of the lesion with relative preservation of vibration and proprioception, due to lack of involvement of the dorsal columns. Light touch is preserved, though patients often report that touch feels different. When the artery of Adamkiewicz is occluded, the rostral level of the lesion is between T9 and L1. When the anterior spinal artery is directly occluded, a lesion in the upper thoracic or upper lumbar region is more common.

Anterior spinal artery syndrome is differentiated from other causes of myelopathy by the preservation of vibration and proprioception. Also, few other causes of myelopathy present with as abrupt an onset.

*Posterior Spinal Artery Occlusion*
Infarction due to occlusion of the posterior spinal arteries is much less common than infarction due to occlusion of the anterior spinal artery. Posterior spinal artery occlusion presents with loss of vibration and proprioception below the level of the lesion.

### *Hemorrhage*

Arteriovenous malformations and venous angiomas can occur in the spinal column in the subarachnoid space or in the parenchyma of the spinal cord. Symptoms develop because of hemorrhage with subsequent mass effect and infarction; the malformation of Foix–Alajouanine often produces symptoms by thrombosis. Patients present with back pain, weakness of the legs, and sensory symptoms that may be intermittent. Symptoms may develop after trauma or childbirth and may be incorrectly attributed solely to spinal injury. Diagnosis is usually made by MRI.

Aneurysms can occur in the spinal column but are responsible for less than one percent of subarachnoid hemorrhages. Patients present with acute onset of back pain, and the pain quickly extends to involve other spinal regions and the head. When the patient presents obtunded, there may be no clue that the origin was spinal; however, a spinal source should be considered if arteriography is unrevealing.

Spinal epidural and subdural hematomas may occur due to seemingly trivial trauma. Children are more likely to develop hemorrhage in the cervical region, while adults develop hemorrhage in the thoracic and lumbar regions. Patients present with severe spinal pain in the affected region followed by development of motor and sensory symptoms appropriate to the level of the lesion.

Intraparenchymal hemorrhage not due to vascular malformation can develop after spinal injury, and it can present with a central cord syndrome or myelopathy; the location of the lesion is a determinant of the symptoms.

### Lesions at Specific Spinal Levels

Any level of the spinal cord can be affected by disease, but the common causes differ at various levels of the neuraxis. For example, cervical myelopathy is commonly due to disk disease and spondylosis, whereas these are uncommon causes of myelopathy in the thoracic regions. In the thoracic regions, the clinician should more readily suspect other pathology, such as tumors. Disorders of the individual nerve roots, including cervical and lumbar radiculopathy, are discussed in Chapter 5.

#### *Craniocervical Junction Lesions*

Craniocervical junction lesions present with varied symptoms and signs depending on the severity of the lesions. Mild disease presents with gait difficulty and sensory loss that is most prominent across the shoulders and extends to the upper arms; dysesthesias extending to the hand can occur.

More severe disease produces quadriparesis with spasticity and sphincter dysfunction, palsies of cranial nerve (CN) IX to CN XII, and downbeat nystagmus. Dysfunction of higher cervical roots produces weakness of paraspinal muscles that, in conjunction with accessory palsy, can produce impairment of head posture.

Common causes of craniocervical junction lesions include tumors at the craniocervical junction and subluxation or fracture of C1. Differential diagnosis includes cervical cord and brain stem lesions. Cord lesions do not produce palsies of the lower cranial nerves. Lower cervical cord lesions spare proximal upper extremity motor function and do not affect phrenic nerve function. Brain stem lesions typically produce alterations in consciousness, except for the locked-in syndrome; in craniocervical lesions, the deficits in CN VII and CN VI nerve function are evident.

## Cervical Cord

### Central Cord Syndrome

Central cord syndrome is usually due to trauma, although it can be due to intrinsic lesions of the cord, including tumors and syringomyelia. When due to trauma, it is usually from hyperextension of the neck. The patient presents with weakness of the arms with relative preservation of the legs, which is so-called man-in-a-barrel syndrome. Some degree of quadriparesis is almost always present, however, including hyperreflexia and upward plantar responses in the legs. The reflexes may be depressed in the arms, especially early in the course. Pain in the hands and arms is common and may be severe.

The clinical findings of central cord syndrome are probably due to damage to the central gray matter. Quadriparesis suggests damage to the lateral corticospinal tracts. There may be dissociated sensory loss in the arms; that is, there may be a deficit in pain and temperature sensation with preservation of touch, vibration, and proprioception. This combination occurs because of involvement of the crossing axons of the anterolateral tracts.

### Cervical Spondylosis

Spondylosis is growth of osteophytes resulting in ankylosis, or loss of mobility, of the spine. Encroachment on the spinal canal produces damage to segmental nerve roots and compression to the spinal cord. Neurologic symptoms can be from radiculopathy due to damage to individual nerve roots at affected levels or from myelopathy due to damage to descending tracts.

Cervical spondylosis is most common at the C5–6 level, with less common involvement at the C6–7 and C4–5 levels. C5–6 spondylosis results in weakness and atrophy of muscles innervated by these roots, especially the biceps and deltoid. Biceps reflex is usually depressed; if there is myelopathy, reflexes below this level will be brisk with upward plantar responses. Corticospinal tract dysfunction often produces incoordination of the hands.

Differential diagnosis of cervical spondylosis includes other causes of myelopathy including tumors. ALS is commonly mistaken for cervical spondylosis with myelopathy, since ALS frequently presents with weakness of the hands and corticospinal tracts in the legs. Many patients with ALS undergo imaging studies of the cervical spine to rule out spondylosis. A differentiating feature is the prominent wasting of intrinsic muscles of the hand seen in most ALS patients; this finding is distinctly absent in cervical spondylosis, which rarely affects C8 and T1 nerve roots. However, if there is any doubt as to the correct diagnosis, imaging should be done, since cervical spondylosis is potentially treatable.

### Thoracic Cord

Causes of lesions in the thoracic region include vascular occlusion, tumors, disk disease, trauma, transverse myelitis, multiple sclerosis, and abscess. Pain as an early symptom suggests an extrinsic lesion producing cord compression while absence of pain suggests an intrinsic lesion, whether neoplastic or inflammatory. The anterior spinal artery syndrome is the most common vascular lesion in the thoracic cord.

Lesions of the upper thoracic cord may have few findings other than those that would help define a sensory level, along with corticospinal tract signs when white matter tracts are affected. Lesions of the lower thoracic cord, especially below T9, may preserve function of the upper abdominal muscles; this condition can result in rostral movement of the umbilicus with a sit-up maneuver (Beevor's sign). Testing of the abdominal reflexes can be helpful in these cases.

### Lumbar Cord

The most common lesions affecting the lumbar cord region are lumbar radiculopathy and spinal stenosis. Tumors and other compressive lesions can affect the cauda equina and conus medullaris.

#### Lumbar Spondylosis and Spinal Stenosis

Spondylosis develops in the lumbar area, just as it does in the cervical spinal cord. Degenerative changes include osteophyte formation, hypertrophy of the posterior ligaments, disk protrusion, and facet hypertrophy. Spondylolisthesis is forward slippage of a vertebral body on the bone beneath; the defect can be degenerative or congenital.

Spinal stenosis is characterized by reduced caliber of the spinal canal, usually due to severe degenerative changes. Spondylosis, ligamentum flavum hypertrophy, and disk protrusion encroach on the subarachnoid space. Patients present with back pain, often exacerbated by walking; patients also complain of leg pain with walking. The spinal claudication is probably due to direct nerve compression plus ischemia of the lower cord and/or nerve roots, since ambulation causes venous engorgement, resulting in reduced effective caliber of the canal and resultant increased compression of the vascular and neural elements.

Diagnosis of spinal stenosis is confirmed by MRI, computerized tomography (CT), or myelography of the lumbar spine. Post-myelography CT scanning can clearly demonstrate the absence of subarachnoid space at affected levels.

An important differential diagnosis is vascular claudication of the legs, since both spinal stenosis and vascular claudication can give pain with walking. No clinical features are diagnostic but there are some general guidelines. Spinal stenosis is suggested by the following:

- Pain most prominent in the thigh
- Neurologic symptoms with exertion, including weakness and dysesthesias
- Improvement over at least several minutes during sitting—but not during standing—after cessation of exertion
- Positional nature of exertional pain—for instance, greater difficulty walking downhill than uphill, little difficulty bicycling
- Stooped posture (not invariably found)
- Peripheral pulses usually present

Vascular claudication is suggested by the following:

- Pain most prominent in the calf
- No or only vague neurologic symptoms with exertion
- Improvement within seconds to a few minutes after cessation of exertion; sitting usually not required

- No positional nature of exertional pain
- Peripheral pulses usually absent

*Cauda Equina and Conus Medullaris Lesions*

The cauda equina (literally, "horse's tail") consists of the lower lumbar and sacral nerve roots. Lesions of the cauda equina produce asymmetric pain and sensory loss in the caudal roots; most symptoms are due to dysfunction of L4 to S2. The ankle tendon reflex is commonly absent. Bowel and bladder symptoms develop with severe disease. Important lesions affecting the cauda equina are lumbar disk disease and spondylosis, ependymoma, metastatic tumors, and trauma with subluxation.

The conus medullaris is the terminal portion of the spinal cord; it is the origination of the most caudal nerve roots. Patients present with bowel and bladder dysfunction early in the disease, whereas these symptoms develop later in cauda equina lesions. Sensory loss in the perineal region may develop. Involvement of the conus medullaris may produce corticospinal tract signs including upward plantar response and hyperreflexia of the Achilles tendon reflex; at the same time, weakness of distal muscles and loss of knee reflexes suggest a lower motoneuron lesion. Important lesions affecting the conus medullaris are the same as those affecting the cauda equina.

*Sacral Cord*

S1 is the sacral root most commonly damaged by degenerative disease of the lumbar spine. Patients present with weakness of the gastrocnemius and intrinsic muscles of the feet. Sensory loss affects the sole of the foot.

S2 lesion produces weakness, which is most prominent in the intrinsic muscles of the feet, but it may be subtle. Sensory loss affects the saddle area.

Lower sacral lesions are rare; they may be caused by trauma or tumors involving the sacrum. Bowel and bladder symptoms and impotence predominate; there are no leg symptoms or signs.

# 5

# Peripheral Nerve and Muscle

## ANATOMY

The essential features of the neuromuscular axis are motor nerves, sensory nerves, autonomic nerves, muscle fibers, and the neuromuscular junction. Nerves are surrounded by processes of Schwann cells, which form myelin sheaths around the nerves.

Motor neurons originate in the spinal cord and brain stem and innervate skeletal muscle (Figure 5.1). Each motor neuron innervates many muscle fibers, but each muscle fiber is innervated by only one motor neuron. The innervation ratio is the number of muscle fibers innervated by a single motor neuron for a particular muscle; the innervation ratio is lowest for extraocular muscles and greatest for large antigravity muscles. The inset of Figure 5.1 shows a diagrammatic representation of a motor nerve innervating a muscle fiber. With denervation, there is loss of motor axons, so surviving axons sprout processes to innervate the denervated muscle fibers; this process increases the innervation ratio.

The neuromuscular junction transduces action potentials of the motor nerves into muscle fiber action potentials. Acetylcholine (ACh) is released by the presynaptic terminal when it is depolarized. The ACh crosses the synaptic cleft and binds to ACh receptors (AChRs); this binding causes channels to open and allows ionic flux in and out of the cell. The preponderance of ionic flux is sodium into the cell, which depolarizes the muscle fiber membrane to the point that it reaches threshold; a muscle fiber action potential is then produced.

The muscle fiber membrane conducts action potentials to the T-tubule system, which triggers release of calcium ($Ca^{++}$) from the sarcoplasmic reticulum. Calcium binds to troponin, producing a con-

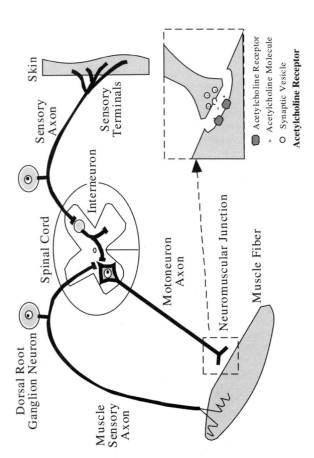

**Fig. 5.1** Diagram of segmental peripheral nerve anatomy shows the motor system on the left side and the sensory system on the right. Central reflex pathways and descending axons are not shown. The inset shows the neuromuscular junction, with release of acetylcholine from the motor axon terminal.

formational change in the actin and allowing interaction with myosin, thereby producing muscle shortening.

Normally, each motor neuron action potential produces one action potential in each of its muscle fibers. Many disorders interfere with this one-to-one transmission: not only disorders of the neuromuscular junction, but also of peripheral nerve and muscle. Most disorders cause failure of muscle fiber potential generation, although a few (for instance, myotonia) cause repetitive discharge of muscle fibers innervated by a single axon.

Sensory neurons have cell bodies in the dorsal root ganglia or sensory ganglia of the cranial nerves. Most sensory neurons are bipolar, with peripheral projections transducing sensory input into action potentials and central projections conducting action potentials to the spinal cord and brain stem. Figure 5.1 (above) shows sensory nerve endings and their projections through afferent nerve fibers.

## EXAMINATION

Examination of the neuromuscular axis includes the following:

- Muscle strength and tone
- Sensory function, including areas of increased and decreased sensitivity to touch, pressure, pain, joint position, vibration, and thermal sensation
- Station and gait
- Tendon reflexes

Muscle strength is graded according to the following scale:

| | |
|---|---|
| 5/5 | Normal |
| 4/5 | Weak but able to move against resistance |
| 3/5 | Able to move against gravity but not resistance |
| 2/5 | Able to move joint but not against gravity |
| 1/5 | Unable to move joint but muscle contraction visible |
| 0/5 | No perceptible muscle contraction |

The span of muscle strength rating 4/5 is huge, necessitating subclassifications such as $4^+/5$, $4^-/5$. Since 5 is, by definition, normal, use of $5^-/5$ is discouraged.

Reflexes are graded according to the following scale:

4/2  Clearly hyperactive, often with clonus
3/2  Brisk but not clearly pathologic
2/2  Normal
1/2  Depressed
0/2  Absent

Hyperactive reflexes indicate an upper motoneuron lesion, hyperadrenergic state, or hyperthyroidism. Neuromuscular disorders preserve reflexes unless the loss of strength is severe, at which point reflexes are suppressed. Sensory neuropathies and demyelinating neuropathies depress reflexes more than other neuromuscular disorders do.

Obviously, a detailed examination could be inordinately lengthy, so the examination is focused based on history and other findings. For example, if a patient appears to have a median neuropathy, the strength of each of the median, ulnar, and radial innervated muscles would be tested; however, the muscles of the leg would be spared a detailed examination, although testing of lower extremity tendon and plantar reflexes could be helpful to rule out a cervical cord lesion. If no signs point to a specific neuromuscular deficit—for instance, if the patient presents with only a headache—I examine the following:

- Strength and tone of deltoid, biceps, triceps, wrist extensors, finger flexors, hand intrinsic muscles, hip flexors, quadriceps, hamstrings, foot dorsiflexors (extensors), and hallux extensors; ability to walk on the ball of the foot reveals normal foot flexor strength
- Sensation to sharp stimulus and vibration distally on each extremity
- Tendon reflexes of the biceps, triceps, quadriceps (patellar tendon), and gastrocnemius (Achilles)
- Gait under the following circumstances: normal, tandem (heel–toe), heel, and toe (actually, ball of the foot).

If the findings of this examination are completely normal and the patient has no neuromuscular complaints, the chance of an undiagnosed neuromuscular condition is small.

## DIFFERENTIAL DIAGNOSIS OF NEUROMUSCULAR DISORDERS

The first task of diagnosing a neuromuscular disorder is to rule out a lesion of the spinal cord and/or brain. Central disorders producing peripheral manifestations usually affect systems other than the peripheral nervous system or have an anatomic distribution that would be unusual with a peripheral lesion. For example, weakness in a left median distribution would suggest a peripheral lesion. Weakness in a median and ulnar distribution would suggest a single lesion at the level of the brachial plexus or higher. If the ipsilateral leg is also weak, a single lesion would have to be in the central nervous system (CNS). Differential diagnosis of neuromuscular disorders depends on detailed anatomical localization, which requires distinguishing among lesions of the following locations:

- Muscle
- Nerve
- Neuromuscular junction

Disorders of muscle and neuromuscular junction produce pure motor symptoms. The only nerve disorders that produce pure motor symptoms are the motor neuron diseases and multifocal motor neuropathy. Reflexes are commonly preserved in disorders of muscle and the neuromuscular junction, unless the weakness is severe. Severe hyporeflexia or areflexia suggests neuropathy and is most common in sensory neuropathy.

### Nerve Conduction Velocity and Electromyography Interpretation

Nerve conduction velocity (NCV) and electromyography (EMG) aid with the differential diagnosis by classifying the neuromuscular defect, first by differentiating muscle from nerve from neuromuscular junction dysfunction (Table 5.1). For patients with neuropathy,

**Table 5.1    Neurodiagnostic Findings with Neuromuscular Lesions**

| Lesion | CMAP | SNAP | Motor NCV | Sensory NCV | EMG |
|---|---|---|---|---|---|
| Motor neuronopathy | Reduced | Normal | Normal or near normal | Normal | Denervation seen |
| Sensory neuronopathy | Normal | Low amplitude | Normal | Mild slowing or absent response | Normal |
| Axonopathy | Reduced | Reduced or absent | Normal or near normal | Normal or near normal | Denervation seen |
| Demyelinating neuropathy | Dispersed | Dispersed or absent | Slow; conduction block | Slow or absent | Normal or denervation seen |
| Myopathy | Normal; possible low amplitude | Normal | Normal | Normal | Myopathic pattern seen |
| Neuromuscular transmission defect | Normal or low amplitude | Normal | Normal | Normal | Normal or myopathic pattern seen |

CMAP = compound motor action potential; SNAP = sensory nerve action potential; NCV = nerve conduction velocity; EMG = electromyography.

the studies can differentiate axonal from demyelinating syndromes and determine which nerves are affected.

Neuropathy typically produces slowing of peripheral nerve conduction velocity and/or reduced amplitude of the compound motor action potential (CMAP) and sensory nerve action potential (SNAP). With chronic denervation, EMG shows fibrillation potentials and positive sharp waves due to spontaneous action potentials in denervated muscle fibers, as well as large-amplitude polyphasic motor unit potentials indicative of reinnervation of muscle fibers by surviving motor axons. Acutely, EMG may only show reduced numbers of functioning units. Neuropathy may be characterized by degeneration mostly of axons, neuron cell bodies, or myelin sheath; this characteristic is discussed below.

Myopathy produces normal nerve conductions, except that the CMAP may be reduced because of the reduced number of muscle fibers activated by the action potentials. Motor unit potentials are small for the same reason, and they are often polyphasic because of dispersed action potential activation and propagation in the muscle fiber membrane; this combination is often called the "brief, small-amplitude polyphasic potential."

Neuromuscular transmission defects have normal NCVs except for reduction of CMAP amplitude, especially in myasthenic syndrome. Repetitive stimulation produces a changing CMAP; the effect of repetitive stimulation differs with individual disorders and stimulation frequency (discussed later).

## Muscle and Nerve Biopsy

Muscle biopsy is indicated for patients in whom the following diagnoses are suspected:

- Muscular dystrophy
- Inflammatory myopathy (polymyositis, dermatomyositis, or infectious or parasitic myopathy)
- Mitochondrial myopathy
- Glycogen and lipid storage disorders
- Vasculitis

Muscle biopsy shows infiltration in most patients with inflammatory myopathies. Dermatomyositis classically features atrophy of the fibers at the periphery of the fascicles, individual fibers undergoing degeneration and regeneration, and perivascular inflammation; however, dermatomyositis may sometimes *not* show such classic features. Muscular dystrophies are characterized by degenerating and regenerating muscle fibers and replacement of muscle tissue by connective tissue. Sural nerve biopsy is indicated for patients in whom the following diagnoses are suspected:

- Vasculitis
- Some demyelinating neuropathies
- Amyloidosis
- Some familial and suspected metabolic neuropathies

For individuals with storage disorders, assays for specific enzymes may be revealing. Focal regions of vascular inflammation suggest vasculitis. Leprosy shows infiltration of white blood cells into nerve segments, and the bacteria may be demonstrated on special stains.

## Laboratory Tests

Creatine kinase (CK) is elevated in most patients with inflammatory myopathy, and it is modestly elevated in some patients with denervating diseases. CK is normal in most neuropathies and in all predominantly sensory neuropathies. CK is often normal in metabolic myopathies. Duchenne muscular dystrophy is associated with a marked elevation in CK, but the increase may be less marked or absent in other dystrophies. Aldolase is also increased in many myopathies; it is less increased in other neuromuscular conditions.

Laboratory tests depend on the type of neuropathy, although many clinicians perform a general battery of tests without regard to the type of neuropathy. The following list of tests may be adapted to the specific type of neuropathy.

- Chemistries
- Complete blood count
- Vitamin $B_{12}$ and folate levels
- Thyroid function (free T4 and thyroid-stimulating hormone)
- Rapid plasma reagin (RPR)
- Twenty-four-hour urine for heavy metals
- Serum protein electrophoresis, serum immunoelectrophoresis, and urine immunoelectrophoresis

Depending on clinical findings, additional tests may be indicated, including human immunodeficiency virus (HIV), red cell cholinesterase, blood lead, lactate, antinuclear antibody (ANA), erythrocyte sedimentation rate, and others. Clinicians should ideally first classify the neuropathy and then judiciously select tests to look for disorders that produce that type of neuropathy.

## NEUROPATHIES

Localization and diagnosis of some important neuropathies are presented in this section. A more comprehensive list of neuropathies is included in the Appendix in Tables A.5 through A.7.

### Differential Diagnosis

Anatomic localization of the lesion in patients with neuropathy is critical to the differential diagnosis. With characterization of the neuropathy, the list of possible diagnoses is narrowed. For example, a subacute demyelinating sensorimotor polyneuropathy would be most suggestive of Guillain–Barré syndrome. A chronic pure motor neuronopathy would be most suggestive of amyotrophic lateral sclerosis or spinal muscular atrophy. Neuropathy should be classified according to the following criteria:

- Modality: motor, sensory, autonomic, or a combination
- Chronicity: acute, subacute, or chronic
- Pathology: neuronal, axonal, or demyelinating
- Distribution: focal, multifocal, or generalized
- Age of onset

Table 5.2 lists some important neuromuscular disorders and their classification according to this scheme.

### *Modality*

Modalities include motor, sensory, and autonomic function. This discussion focuses on motor and sensory function. The most common neuropathies are sensorimotor, indicating damage to peripheral nerves without preference to modality. Pure motor or sensory neuropathies are usually due to direct neuronal damage at the soma—that is, at the motoneurons (anterior horn cells) or dorsal root ganglion neurons, respectively.

Motor neuropathies are characterized clinically by weakness often with fasciculations and muscle cramps. NCV testing shows

**Table 5.2 Important Neuropathies and Neuronopathies**

| Disorder | Chro-nicity | Distribu-tion | Modality | Pathology |
|---|---|---|---|---|
| Amyotrophic lateral sclerosis | C | G | M | A |
| Carpal tunnel syndrome | C | F | SM | A, D |
| CIDP | C | G | SM | D |
| Conduction block neuropathy | C | M | M, SM | D |
| Diabetic neuropathy | C | G, M, F | S, SM | A |
| Guillain–Barré syndrome | A or S | G | SM | D |
| Spinal muscular atrophy | C | G | M | A |

CIDP = chronic inflammatory demyelinating polyradiculoneuropathy; Chronicity: C = chronic; A = acute; S = subacute; Distribution: G = generalized; F = focal; M = multifocal; Modality: M = motor; S = sensory; SM = sensorimotor; Pathology: A = axonal or neuronal; D = demyelinating.

low-amplitude CMAPs and occasionally reduced motor NCVs, depending on pathology. EMG shows denervation in affected muscles. Polyneuropathies usually affect distal muscles more than proximal muscles.

Sensory neuropathies are characterized clinically by loss of sensation and presence of abnormal sensations. Paresthesias are abnormal spontaneous sensory perceptions, such as tingling. Dysesthesias are abnormal perceptions of sensory stimuli, as when a pressure sensation induces tingling or pain. If large-diameter axons are involved in the neuropathy, the abnormal sensation is commonly tingling, while if small fibers are predominantly involved, the sensation is often burning. NCV testing in pure sensory neuropathies shows reduced SNAP amplitude and often slow sensory NCV, depending on pathology. EMG shows no denervation in muscle.

Sensorimotor neuropathies are characterized by the combined symptoms of motor and sensory neuropathies; however, fasciculations are unusual. NCV testing shows low-amplitude CMAPs and

SNAPs with moderate to severe axonal neuropathies. Demyelinating neuropathies produce slow motor and sensory NCVs and have focal areas of conduction block early in the course.

Autonomic neuropathies are characterized clinically by vasomotor and gastrointestinal motility dysfunction; the most common effects are orthostatic hypotension and gastroparesis. Conventional NCV testing and EMG show no abnormalities unless sensory neuropathy and motor neuropathy coexist. Special studies of sympathetic function can reveal the dysfunction.

### Chronicity

Most neuropathies are chronic. Neurotoxins tend to produce CNS symptoms acutely, with neuropathy as a delayed effect that often appears only after prolonged exposure.

Acute neuropathies are predominantly mononeuropathies, such as pressure palsies and nerve infarctions. Guillain–Barré syndrome (GBS) has been described as acute; however, the onset is typically subacute. Other subacute neuropathies include diphtheric neuropathy, diabetic amyotrophy, and porphyria.

### Pathology

Pathology reveals the type of neuropathy. There are three basic types: axonal, neuronal, and demyelinating. This classification scheme has different significance than the tripartite classification of extent of damage of neurapraxia, axonotmesis, and neurotmesis. Neurapraxia is traumatic disruption of nerve fiber function without transection of axons. Axonotmesis is traumatic breakage of axons with an intact connective tissue sheath. Neurotmesis is complete transection of the nerve.

Axonal neuropathies are due to degeneration of the axons and form the largest group of neuropathies. Longer axons are affected more severely, so the symptoms and signs are more prominent distally. No symptoms are particularly distinctive for axonal neuropathy; differentiation from demyelination is made predominantly on the basis of NCV testing and EMG. Examination reveals preserved deep tendon reflexes (DTRs) in patients with axonal neuropathies, in contrast to the depressed reflexes seen with demyelinating neuropathies. Muscle weakness is accompanied by muscle atrophy, which is more prominent with increasing chronicity.

Neuronopathies are due to degeneration of the nerve cell body and imply a metabolic or genetic defect. Since the motoneurons and dorsal root ganglion neurons are usually not directly affected by the same pathological process, the symptoms will be motor or sensory, depending on the neurons involved. Neuronopathies are difficult to distinguish clinically from axonopathies. Features that would suggest a neuronopathy include involvement of a single modality, fasciculations, reduced CMAP or SNAP with normal NCV, and denervation of distal *and* very proximal muscles, such as the paraspinals.

Demyelinating neuropathies are characterized clinically by motor and sensory symptoms, especially weakness, paresthesias, dysesthesias, and sensory loss. Symptoms may be both proximal and distal, although distal musculature is predominantly affected. Demyelinating neuropathies often lack the distal symmetric ascending character of axonal neuropathies. Examination shows depressed DTRs; for example, the diagnosis of GBS is doubtful if DTRs are preserved, even early in the course. Depressed DTRs are the main differentiating feature from axonal and neuronal degenerations, and if the DTRs are depressed out of proportion to the weakness, a demyelinating neuropathy is suspected. Motor and sensory NCVs are slow. CMAPs and SNAPs are low in amplitude with a dispersed waveform, in contrast to low-amplitude preserved waveshape seen in axonal neuropathies. Demyelinating neuropathies frequently produce prominent weakness with unimpressive atrophy compared with that seen in axonal neuropathies.

### Distribution

Neuropathies are focal, multifocal, or generalized. Patients with generalized neuropathies are predisposed to develop pressure palsies, which present as focal neuropathies; in these cases, common damaged areas are the median nerve at the carpal tunnel, the ulnar nerve at the ulnar groove, and the peroneal nerve at the fibular neck.

Multifocal neuropathies are usually due to a systemic disorder. Important causes include diabetes, leprosy, polyarteritis nodosa, and other vasculitides. Familial predisposition to pressure palsies may also present with the symptoms of mononeuropathy multiplex.

Generalized neuropathies usually have a distal predominance, although examination, NCV testing, and EMG reveal both proximal and distal damage. Because of the distal symptoms, upper extremity dysfunction may be revealed only on NCV testing and EMG.

### *Age of Onset*

Many neuropathies that occur in adults do not occur in children. For example, a chronic pure motor neuronopathy in an adult would most likely be amyotrophic lateral sclerosis (ALS), but in children it would more likely be spinal muscular atrophy (SMA). SMA can occur later in life but only rarely does. The presence of signs of upper motor neuron involvement would add more security to the diagnosis of ALS. Important neuropathies and neuronopathies in children include the following:

- Spinal muscular atrophy
- Metabolic disorders (for instance, storage disease)
- Juvenile diabetes
- Vincristine neuropathy in children with certain cancers
- Guillain–Barré syndrome
- Hereditary neuropathies

### Polyneuropathies

The most important differentiating feature in polyneuropathies is between axonal and demyelinating. Most metabolic neuropathies are axonal, including diabetes, renal neuropathy, and most drug-induced neuropathies. Demyelinating neuropathies are more rare and include the immune-mediated neuropathies.

### Diabetic Neuropathy

Common types of diabetic neuropathy include the following:

- Sensorimotor axonal neuropathy
- Mononeuropathy
- Mononeuropathy multiplex
- Diabetic polyradiculopathy
- Sensory neuropathy
- Autonomic neuropathy

Mononeuropathies due to diabetes mellitus include cranial nerve palsies, especially of cranial nerve (CN) III and CN VI. These are discussed in Chapter 3.

#### Sensorimotor Neuropathy

Diabetic sensorimotor neuropathy is an axonal degeneration indistinguishable clinically from the multitude of other axonal sensorimotor neuropathies. Diabetes is by far the most common cause of axonal neuropathy in the United States. Distal numbness in a stocking and glove distribution is present early in the course. Weakness develops later and involves distal muscles, especially intrinsic muscles of the feet, tibialis anterior, and hands.

#### Mononeuropathy Multiplex

Diabetes is the most common cause of mononeuropathy multiplex. The ulnar nerve is commonly affected, producing wasting of ulnar-innervated intrinsic muscles of the hand and numbness of digit 5 and the ulnar half of digit 4. Median and peroneal nerves are also commonly affected. Cranial neuropathies include oculomotor palsy (see Chapter 3).

#### Sensory Neuropathy

Diabetic sensory neuropathy mostly affects predominantly unmyelinated C fibers and small myelinated fibers, which subserve pain and temperature sensation and, to a lesser extent, light touch. Symptoms include a burning pain distally. Feet are affected first; the pain later ascends, and the hands may be affected. Patients notice the pain especially at night when trying to sleep. Examination shows increased threshold for touch stimuli; stimuli, when perceived, are often painful. Vibration and proprioception are unaffected early in the course, but they are eventually lost. NCV testing shows preserved motor and sensory NCVs early in the course, but the size of the SNAP is reduced. Later, the sensory NCV is slowed, and the SNAP ultimately disappears. Motor NCV eventually slows since the diabetic "sensory neuropathy" is really a sensorimotor axonal neuropathy with predominantly sensory features.

*Diabetic Polyradiculopathy*

Patients present with pain, sensory loss, and muscle weakness appropriate to the level of involvement. When involvement is in the upper lumbar region, the clinical syndrome of diabetic amyotrophy is produced. Pain is in the low back and upper legs, and there is weakness of the quadriceps and psoas, along with a reduced quadriceps reflex. Sensory loss is in the L2–4 distribution, although the dysesthetic pain may overshadow the heightened sensory threshold. Direct involvement of the femoral nerve has been implicated by some investigators.

Diabetic radiculopathy may occur in the thoracic dermatomes, often triggering extensive evaluation for spinal lesions. Because of the important differential diagnoses of herniated disk, spinal tumor, and degenerative disease, magnetic resonance imaging of the affected area often has to be performed.

### Guillain–Barré Syndrome

GBS is also known as "acute inflammatory demyelinating polyradiculoneuropathy." It affects Schwann cells, producing demyelination of peripheral nerves. Proximal myelin segments are affected first. Patients present with generalized weakness, which usually spares the extraocular muscles. Facial weakness may be prominent. Sensory symptoms include numbness that spans sensory modalities and is most prominent distally. Reflexes are almost always absent, even early in the course.

Motor and sensory NCVs are slow and the waveforms have a dispersed appearance—that is, they have a lower amplitude and longer duration, indicating that there is increased variance in conduction velocity. However, in patients with very early disease,

NCVs may be normal. F waves are absent or markedly delayed in almost all patients, and they are abnormal before distal peripheral nerve conduction is affected. EMG shows reduced motor unit recruitment; subsequent axonal degeneration produces fibrillation potentials, although this is uncommon early in the course. Cerebrospinal fluid (CSF) in GBS has high protein with few or no white blood cells (WBCs).

The axonal variety of GBS is a rare condition that presents with similar symptoms and signs, but neurophysiological studies show mostly axonal degeneration with less impressive demyelination.

Differential diagnosis of GBS includes other causes of subacute weakness, such as tick paralysis, acute porphyria, botulism, hypophosphatemia, hypokalemia, and rare toxic neuropathies (caused by, for instance, organophosphate insecticides, *N*-hexane, or arsenic). HIV-associated GBS is of increasing concern.

### Chronic Inflammatory Demyelinating Polyradiculoneuropathy

Chronic inflammatory demyelinating polyradiculoneuropathy (CIDP) is an autoimmune disorder of peripheral nerves. While CIDP is sometimes considered a chronic form of GBS, the immunology may be very different. Patients present with proximal as well as distal weakness, absent reflexes, and distal sensory loss. CSF shows high protein with few or no WBCs. NCV testing shows multifocal slowing with increased latencies of the CMAPs and SNAPs. EMG shows reduced motor unit recruitment early in the course. With secondary axonal degeneration, denervation is seen in the muscles. The differential diagnosis of CIDP includes the hereditary demyelinating neuropathies, paraneoplastic neuropathy, HIV neuropathy, and demyelinating neuropathy with monoclonal gammopathy.

### Hereditary Neuropathies

*Hereditary Motor–Sensory Neuropathy I*

Hereditary motor–sensory neuropathy (HMSN), type I, is also known as the hypertrophic form of Charcot–Marie–Tooth (CMT) disease. It is a demyelinating neuropathy that presents with slowly progressive distal weakness and few sensory symptoms. HMSN I can produce pes cavus deformity of the foot and distal atrophy in the leg, giving a characteristic appearance. Inheritance is autosomal dominant with variable penetrance. Pathology shows demyelinating neuropathy with areas of hypertrophy of the myelin sheath. NCVs are very slow, and EMG usually shows distal denervation, but this is not as prominent as the slowing of the NCVs.

*Hereditary Motor–Sensory Neuropathy II*
HMSN II is also known as the neuronal form of CMT disease. It is an neuronopathy that presents with distal weakness and minimal sensory symptoms. Onset of symptoms is later than with HMSN I. Inheritance is autosomal dominant with variable penetrance. NCVs are near normal but EMG shows prominent denervation.

*Hereditary Motor–Sensory Neuropathy III*
HMSN III is also known as Dejerine–Sottas disease. It is a demyelinating neuropathy with onset in early childhood; patients present with delayed walking and delayed achievement of other motor milestones. Inheritance is autosomal recessive. Infants may present with hypotonia and difficulty feeding; they may be given the diagnosis of congenital hypomyelinating neuropathy. NCVs are very slow and occasionally unobtainable. EMG shows denervation. Pathology shows demyelination or amylenation with hypertrophic changes.

*Hereditary Motor–Sensory Neuropathy IV*
HMSN IV is also known as Refsum disease. It is a rare, predominantly demyelinating neuropathy; it usually presents with retinal degeneration, and the neuropathy is symptomatic only later in the course. Associated symptoms include pigmentary retinal degeneration, ichthyosis, cataracts, and cardiac conduction defects. Inheritance is autosomal recessive; the defect is a deficiency of phytanic acid oxidase. Motor and sensory NCVs are slow.

*Hereditary Sensory Neuropathy*
Hereditary sensory neuropathy is a family of disorders including five entities, all of which are characterized by sensory loss without

motor symptoms. Type I is autosomal dominant, and the remainder are recessive or of uncertain inheritance. Sensory NCVs are slow with reduction in amplitude of the SNAP; SNAP may be unrecordable in many patients. Motor NCVs and CMAPs are normal in most patients, although in type III (familial dysautonomia or Riley–Day syndrome) motor NCVs may be slightly slowed, indicating that type III is a predominantly, though not purely, sensory neuropathy. Many of the sensory neuropathies have autonomic involvement, which manifests as anhidrosis, orthostatic blood pressure, and fluctuating body temperature.

**Mononeuropathies**

Descriptions of mononeuropathies can be voluminous, since almost every nerve in the body has at least one described syndrome. The most common and most important mononeuropathies are discussed here. Upper extremity neuropathies are covered first, lower extremity neuropathies second. Cranial neuropathies are discussed in Chapter 3.

*Cervical Radiculopathy*

The most common cervical root to be damaged is C7, followed by C8, C6, and C5. Most cervical radiculopathies are due to lateral prolapse of the intervertebral disk. Occasionally, osteophytes or spondylitic bars may produce the same effect. Typical clinical findings in common cervical radiculopathies are presented in Table 5.3.

**Table 5.3   Cervical Radiculopathy**

| Root | Sensory Loss | Motor Loss |
|------|--------------|------------|
| C5 | Radial forearm | Deltoid, biceps |
| C6 | Digits 1 and 2 | Biceps, brachioradialis |
| C7 | Digits 3 and 4 | Wrist extensors, triceps |
| C8 | Digit 5 | Intrinsic hand muscles |

**Table 5.4  Clinical Features of Disorders of the Brachial Plexus**

| Disorder | Features |
| --- | --- |
| Brachial plexitis | Usually upper plexus, C5–6, though can be lower; pain initially, followed by arm weakness as pain abates |
| Neoplastic infiltration | Usually lower plexus, C8–T1; painful; lung tumor or lymphoma most common; Horner's syndrome can occur |
| Radiation plexopathy | Usually upper plexus, C5–6; usually painless, uncomfortable dysesthesias sometimes occur |
| Trauma | Any portion of the plexus can be involved |

### Brachial Plexopathy

The most common brachial plexopathies are brachial plexitis, neoplastic infiltration, radiation plexopathy, and trauma. Salient features of each are described in Table 5.4. The brachial plexus is illustrated in Figure 5.2.

### Median Neuropathy

The most common median neuropathy is carpal tunnel syndrome, followed by anterior interosseus syndrome, pronator teres syndrome, and the ligament of Struthers syndrome. Essential features of each are presented in Table 5.5.

### Ulnar Neuropathy

The ulnar nerve is most commonly injured at the elbow, across the ulnar groove and extending into the cubital tunnel. Distal damage to the ulnar nerve can produce varying symptoms and signs; the combination of weakness of the interossei with sparing of the abductor digiti minimi and of sensory function suggests a deep branch lesion in the palm and can be seen in bicycle riders. Compression of the superficial sensory branch may produce sensory symptoms over digit 5 without motor findings. Common ulnar neuropathies are listed in Table 5.6.

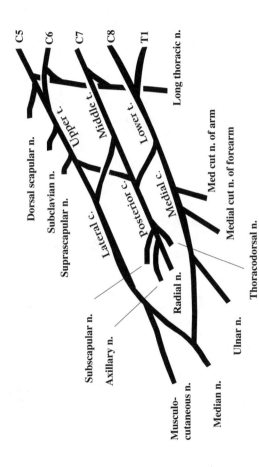

**Fig. 5.2** The roots forming the brachial plexus interconnect and form the major nerves of the arm (n., nerve; cut, cutaneous; med, medial; c., cord; t., trunk).

**Table 5.5    Common Median Neuropathies**

| Disorder | Clinical Findings | Neurodiagnostic Findings |
|---|---|---|
| Carpal tunnel syndrome | Numbness on palmar aspects of digits 1–3; APB weakness when severe | Slow motor and sensory NCVs through tunnel; denervation in APB with severe disease |
| Anterior interosseus syndrome | No sensory loss; weakness of FDP, pronator quadratus, flexor pollicis longus | Denervation in FDP, flexor pollicis longus, and pronator quadratus; APB is normal |
| Pronator teres syndrome | Tenderness over pronator teres; weakness of distal median-innervated muscles | Slow motor NCV through proximal forearm, denervation in muscles distal to pronator teres |
| Ligament of Struthers syndrome | Numbness on palmar hand; weakness of distal median-innervated muscles | As in pronator teres syndrome, plus denervation of pronator teres muscle |

APB = abductor pollicis brevis; FDP = flexor digitorum profundus; NCV = nerve conduction velocity.

### Radial Neuropathy

The most common radial neuropathy is "Saturday night palsy," compression of the radial nerve at the spiral groove of the humerus. It received this name because it typically occurs in patients who rest their arm over a bed or chair when they are deeply asleep, especially when intoxicated. All of the distal radial-innervated muscles in the arm may be affected. The triceps may also be affected if the compression is proximal to its innervation. Patients present with wrist drop and preserved finger flexors and intrinsic muscle strength in the hand. Wrist and finger flexors may appear to be weak if the hand is allowed to fall into a flexed position; the examiner must forcibly extend the wrist to at least the neutral position to accurately test these muscles. Common radial neuropathies are presented in Table 5.7.

**Table 5.6 Common Ulnar Neuropathies**

| Disorder | Clinical Findings | Neurodiagnostic Findings |
|---|---|---|
| Entrapment at or near the elbow* | Numbness over digits 4 and 5 | Slow motor NCV across elbow; denervation in ADM and ulnar half of FDP |
| Entrapment at Guyon's canal | Numbness over digits 4 and 5 and ulnar aspect of hand; dorsal aspect spared | Slow motor and sensory NCV through wrist |
| Lesion of the palmar branch | Weakness of dorsal interossei; no sensory loss | Normal NCV; denervation in first dorsal interosseus but not ADM |
| Lesion of superficial sensory branch | Numbness on dorsal aspect of digit 5 and part of digit 4 | Increased SNAP latency and decreased SNAP amplitude; otherwise normal NCV; no denervation |

ADM = abductor digiti minimi; FDP = flexor digitorum profundus; nerve conduction velocity; SNAP = sensory nerve action potential.

*Includes tardy ulnar palsy and cubital tunnel syndrome.

**Table 5.7 Common Radial Neuropathies**

| Disorder | Clinical Findings | Neurodiagnostic Findings |
|---|---|---|
| Compression at spiral groove | Weakness of finger and wrist extensor; triceps spared; sensory loss on dorsal surface of the thumb (often subtle) | Slow motor NCV across spiral groove; denervation in distal radial-innervated muscles; triceps may be affected with proximal lesions |
| Posterior interosseus syndrome | Weakness of finger and wrist extensors; no sensory loss | Denervation in wrist and finger extensors; supinator and extensor carpi radialis longus spared |

NCV = nerve conduction velocity.

### *Lumbosacral Radiculopathy*

Lumbosacral radiculopathy typically produces back pain radiating down the leg in a distribution appropriate to the involved nerve root. Table 5.8 presents symptoms typically seen with radiculopathy at various levels.

The most common lumbosacral radiculopathy is L5 to S1 with entrapment of the S1 nerve root. In addition to the sensory and motor findings, the Achilles tendon reflex is often absent. EMG shows denervation in affected muscles, and the H-reflex is usually absent.

The second most common lumbar radiculopathy involves the L5 nerve root; it is caused by impingement at L4–5. There are no reflex abnormalities. Weakness of the peroneus longus and tibialis anterior muscles is very helpful for this diagnosis. Examination of the tibialis posterior action can differentiate between L5 radiculopathy and peroneal neuropathy, since this muscle is innervated by a branch of the tibial nerve.

### *Lumbosacral Plexopathy*

The most common causes of lumbosacral plexopathy is neoplastic infiltration from paravertebral metastases and local extension of ab-

**Table 5.8   Lumbosacral Radiculopathy**

| Root | Sensory Loss | Motor Loss | Reflex Abnormality |
|------|-------------|-----------|--------------------|
| L2 | Lateral and anterior upper thigh | Psoas, quadriceps | None |
| L3 | Lower medial thigh | Psoas, quadriceps | Patellar tendon |
| L4 | Medial lower leg | Tibialis anterior, quadriceps | Patellar tendon |
| L5 | Lateral lower leg | Peroneus longus, gluteus medius, tibialis anterior, toe extension | None |
| S1 | Lateral foot; digits 4 and 5; outside of sole | Gastrocnemius, gluteus maximus | Achilles tendon |

dominal tumors, such as gastrointestinal and renal tumors. Lumbar plexitis is rare, and its course and presentation parallel those of brachial plexitis. Patients with lumbar plexopathy present with weakness spanning single dermatomal or neural distributions, such as quadriceps and adductors. NCVs are usually normal. EMG can show denervation, but it is frequently normal if performed early in the course. The lumbosacral plexus is illustrated in Figure 5.3.

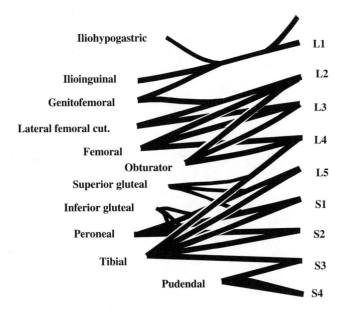

**Fig. 5.3** The roots forming the lumbosacral plexus interconnect, forming the major nerves of the abdomen and leg (cut., cutaneous).

### Sciatic Neuropathy

Injury to the sciatic nerve usually occurs where it exits the pelvis. Typical causes include intramuscular injections, pelvic fractures, blunt trauma to the buttock or posterior thigh, and stretch from trauma or surgery.

The peroneal division is more susceptible to traumatic injury than the tibial division; therefore, some sciatic neuropathies are misinterpreted as peroneal nerve palsies. Patients present with weakness of the tibialis anterior. Weakness of the gastrocnemius is difficult to assess because of the tremendous strength of this muscle even in small individuals; the proportionate weakness required for the deficit to be detectable is large.

### Peroneal Neuropathy

Peroneal neuropathy is most often due to compression of the nerve at the fibular neck. Damage to the peroneal division of the sciatic nerve may produce similar symptoms. Patients present with weakness of the tibialis anterior and peroneii, producing impaired dorsiflexion and eversion of the foot. NCV is slowed across the fibular neck. EMG shows denervation in the tibialis anterior and peroneus longus. Differentiation of peroneal neuropathy across the fibular neck from a more proximal peroneal lesion is accomplished by EMG of the short head of the biceps femoris; this muscle is innervated by a branch of the peroneal division after it has separated from the tibial division but before it has passed through the popliteal fossa.

### Tibial Neuropathy

Tibial neuropathy is uncommon and usually traumatic; gunshot wounds, needle injections, and motor vehicle accidents with leg fractures are frequent causes. Most patients with proximal tibial neuropathy also have dysfunction of the peroneal division. Patients present with weakness of the gastrocnemius and soleus muscles, which manifests as an inability to stand on the toes or, minimally, relative weakness of plantar flexion.

Tarsal tunnel syndrome is an uncommon problem; it occurs due to entrapment of a distal branch of the tibial nerve as it passes behind the medial malleolus. Patients present with pain and dysesthesias in the foot and with tenderness in the region of entrapment. NCV shows slowing of conduction in the medial and lateral plantar nerves, the terminal branches of the tibial nerve. EMG may show denervation in the abductor hallucis and abductor digiti minimi with entrapment of the medial and lateral plantar nerves, respectively.

### Femoral Neuropathy

The femoral nerve is injured in the pelvis as it crosses under the inguinal ligament or in the leg. Weakness is most easily detected in the psoas since the quadriceps is so strong. Absent patellar reflex is common. Sensory loss is over the anterior thigh and medial aspect of the calf; this loss in a saphenous nerve distribution is helpful in differentiating femoral neuropathy from lumbar radiculopathy. NCV of the femoral nerve can be done easily in trim individuals but may be impossible in heavier patients. EMG shows denervation of the quadriceps with sparing of adductors (which are innervated by the obturator nerve).

### Lateral Femoral Cutaneous Neuropathy

Entrapment of the lateral femoral cutaneous nerve occurs as it crosses beneath the inguinal ligament. Obesity and pregnancy predispose to this lesion. Patients present with numbness and often pain on the lateral aspect of the thigh. The deficit does not extend below the knee. Lateral femoral cutaneous neuropathy is differentiated from femoral neuropathy by the presence of a lateral sensory deficit and absence of a motor deficit. NCV of this nerve can be reliably performed in trim individuals but may be technically difficult in heavier patients, who are especially prone to lateral femoral cutaneous nerve entrapment.

### Obturator Neuropathy

This very rare condition is usually due to obturator hernia or pelvic fracture. Patients present with weak hip adductors. NCVs are not performed on this nerve. EMG shows denervation in the adductors with preservation of femoral-innervated muscles.

## Mononeuropathy Multiplex

Mononeuropathy multiplex is dysfunction of multiple single peripheral nerves. Coincidental mononeuropathies can occur, but when two or more neuropathies are present, a systemic disorder is usually present. Important causes are diabetes, vasculitides (for instance, polyarteritis nodosa), and leprosy. NCV shows multifocal slowing of nerve conduction in affected nerves.

Classification of mononeuropathy multiplex in the setting of a polyneuropathy is controversial. If the severity of damage to individual nerves far exceeds the NCV and EMG abnormalities due to the polyneuropathy, then the diagnosis of mononeuropathy multiplex is probably reasonable. Some clinicians maintain that, in the presence of a polyneuropathy, multiple mononeuropathies do not have the same pathophysiological and clinical significance.

## Motoneuron Disease

Motoneuron diseases spare sensory nerves and must be distinguished from myopathies, which also only produce motor symptoms. The three most important motoneuron diseases are discussed below.

### Amyotrophic Lateral Sclerosis

In ALS, degeneration of the upper and lower motoneurons develops in midlife or later. Patients present with weakness without sensory loss but with upper motoneuron signs, including hyperreflexia and upward plantar responses. EMG shows widespread fasciculations and denervation.

### Spinal Muscular Atrophy

In SMA, degeneration of lower motoneurons without effect on upper motoneurons begins in utero. Patients present with weakness and hypotonia without sensory or upper motoneuron signs. Late-onset cases of SMA must be distinguished from ALS and muscular dystrophies.

## *Poliomyelitis*

In poliomyelitis, an enterovirus affects the lower motoneuron during an acute illness characterized by malaise, fever, and asymmetric paralysis. The presentation is classic and distinct from that of other motoneuron diseases, but poliomyelitis must be differentiated from GBS and postinfectious encephalomyelitis. EMG shows denervation without sensory nerve involvement and with only mildly slowed motor NCVs, in contrast to findings in GBS (see above).

## *Multifocal Motor Neuropathy*

Multifocal motor neuropathy is easily confused with other motoneuron diseases. Rather than neuronal degeneration, the pathology is multifocal demyelination affecting motor axons. Laboratory tests may show high titers of antibodies to gangliosides. Multifocal motor neuropathy is differentiated from other motoneuron degenerations by NCV and EMG.

## MYOPATHIES

Myopathies present with muscle weakness without sensory dysfunction. Myopathies are differentiated from ALS by the absence of upper motoneuron signs. NCVs are normal in myopathies, although the CMAP may be reduced in muscles with atrophy. EMG in myopathies shows abnormal motor unit potentials that are different from the potentials seen in neuropathies. See Table 5.1 for differentiation of myopathy from neuropathy.

### Dystrophies

Muscular dystrophies are characterized by degeneration of muscle fibers associated with infiltration of connective tissue. The features of the principal dystrophies are presented in Table 5.9.

### Inflammatory Myopathies

Inflammatory myopathies may be autoimmune or infectious. Autoimmune myopathies include polymyositis and dermatomyositis. Polymyositis is classified by whether it is associated with skin

**Table 5.9  Muscular Dystrophies**

| Disorder | Inheritance | Features |
|---|---|---|
| Duchenne MD | X-linked recessive | Weakness, pseudohypertrophy of the calves, Gowers's sign; survival to late adolescence |
| Facioscapulo-humeral MD | Autosomal dominant | Facial weakness followed by arm weakness, scapular winging |
| Humeroperoneal MD (Emery–Dreifuss) | X-linked | Weakness of arms, shoulders, and lower legs in peroneal distribution; contractures of neck, elbows, and ankles; cardiac conduction defects |
| Limb-girdle | Variable | Probably more than one entity, all with arm and shoulder weakness |
| Myotonic MD | Autosomal dominant | Weakness of distal muscles, myotonia, hatchet facies, cataracts, glucose intolerance |
| Ocular MD (may be subset of oculo-pharyngeal MD) | Autosomal dominant | Ptosis progressing to extraocular muscle weakness, occasional facial and other muscle weakness |
| Oculopharyngeal MD | Autosomal dominant | Ptosis, ocular weakness, dysphagia; characteristic muscle biopsy findings |
| Scapuloperoneal MD | Autosomal dominant or X-linked recessive | Foot drop, shoulder weakness; extensor digitorum brevis spared; onset in childhood |

MD = muscular dystrophy.

changes (dermatomyositis) or associated systemic disorders, such as neoplasm or connective tissue disease. Infectious myopathies include a wide range of parasitic, bacterial, and viral infections. Table 5.10 shows the essential features of inflammatory myopathies. Criteria for the diagnosis of polymyositis have been established. Most of the following features must be present for diagnosis:

- Myopathic pattern on EMG
- Perifascicular atrophy, mononuclear infiltration, and degenerating and regenerating muscle fibers on muscle biopsy
- Elevated creatine kinase

Bohan and Peter (NEJM 292:344, 1975) devised a classification scheme for polymyositis and dermatomyositis, as follows:

- Type I: idiopathic polymyositis
- Type II: idiopathic dermatomyositis
- Type III: polymyositis or dermatomyositis associated with cancer
- Type IV: childhood polymyositis or dermatomyositis associated with vasculitis
- Type V: polymyositis or dermatomyositis associated with collagen vascular disease

Viral myositis frequently presents in children with diffuse myalgias. CK is increased but less so than in some other disorders of skeletal muscle.

**Metabolic Myopathies**

Metabolic myopathies result in muscle damage by virtue of either impairment in energy metabolism or abnormal storage of metabolic products that secondarily interfere with muscle metabolism. Table 5.11 shows the clinical features and defects associated with some of the important metabolic myopathies. Muscle biopsy with biochemical analysis of enzyme function is required for diagnosis of most of these disorders.

**Periodic Paralysis**

Periodic paralysis includes a group of disorders characterized by episodic weakness. The exact symptoms and chemistry differ between individual disorders.

Familial hypokalemic periodic paralysis is characterized by attacks of weakness that begin in proximal muscles and spread to distal muscles. An attack can be provoked by rest following intense exercise or by a high-carbohydrate meal and can last up to several hours. Familial hypokalemic periodic paralysis is inherited as

**Table 5.10 Inflammatory Myopathies**

| Disorder | Features |
|---|---|
| Polymyositis in adults | Progressive proximal weakness, elevated CK, myopathic features on EMG, inflammatory infiltrate on muscle biopsy |
| Dermatomyositis in adults | Symptoms of polymyositis with discoloration of eyelids and rash on the dorsum of fingers, especially MCP and PIP joints |
| Childhood inflammatory myopathy with vasculitis | Dermatomyositis common with vasculitic changes on muscle biopsy |
| Polymyositis with connective tissue disorder | Polymyositis in the setting of SLE, RA, and Sjögren's syndrome; arthritis, nephritis, and Raynaud's disease common |
| Inflammatory myopathy with systemic cancer | Polymyositis or dermatomyositis associated with cancer, especially of lung, breast, ovary, stomach |
| Inclusion body myositis | Proximal and distal weakness in adults, usually in older age; findings commonly asymmetric; mild CK elevation; diagnosis by muscle biopsy |
| Polymyalgia rheumatica | Muscle pain and stiffness, usually most prominent in the proximal upper extremity and shoulder girdle muscles; high ESR |
| Viral myositis | Muscle pain; CK elevated |
| Parasitic myositis | Muscle pains with fever and malaise; rare causes are trichinosis, cysticercosis, and toxoplasmosis |
| Bacterial myositis | Muscles hot, swollen, and tender; rarely, Staphylococcus aureus may produce focal or multifocal muscle infections |

CK = creatine kinase; EMG electromyography; MCP = metacarpal; PIP = proximal interphalangeal; SLE = systemic lupus erythematosus; RA = rheumatoid arthritis; ESR = erythrocyte sedimentation rate.

**Table 5.11   Metabolic Myopathies**

| Disorder | Clinical Features | Diagnostic Features |
|---|---|---|
| *Glycogen Storage Diseases* | | |
| Muscle phosphorylase deficiency (McArdle's disease) | Cramps with exercise, myoglobinuria | Phosphorylase deficiency on muscle biopsy; excessive glycogen storage |
| PFK deficiency | Cramps with exercise; autosomal recessive | PFK deficiency on muscle biopsy; excessive glycogen storage |
| Phosphoglycerate kinase deficiency | Cramps with exercise; X-linked recessive | Enzymatic defect on muscle biopsy; no excess glycogen |
| LDH deficiency | Cramps with exercise; autosomal recessive | LDH deficiency on muscle biopsy |
| Acid maltase deficiency (Pompe's disease) | *Infantile onset:* hypotonia, hepatomegaly, death within 2 years; *Adult onset:* progressive weakness and atrophy | Acid maltase deficiency on muscle biopsy; CK elevated; EMG abnormalities sometimes confined to proximal muscles in adult form |
| Debrancher deficiency (Cori's disease) | Weakness and wasting of muscles, multiorgan involvement; autosomal recessive | Enzymatic defect on muscle biopsy; glycogen accumulation in muscle |
| Brancher deficiency | Weakness and wasting; autosomal recessive | Enzymatic defect on muscle biopsy; liver involvement |
| *Lipid Storage Diseases* | | |
| Carnitine deficiency: muscular and systemic | Progressive weakness with bouts of hepatic encephalopathy common in systemic form | Serum carnitine reduced in systemic but not muscle form; muscle biopsy shows reduced carnitine plus abnormal lipid accumulation |
| CPT deficiency | Weakness, painful cramps; myoglobinuria | Decreased CPT on muscle biopsy and in leukocytes |

**Table 5.11** *(continued)*

| Disorder | Clinical Features | Diagnostic Features |
|----------|-------------------|---------------------|
| **Mitochondrial Disorders** | | |
| Kearns–Sayre syndrome | Ophthalmoplegia, ataxia; heart block, retinal degeneration; sporadic | Clinical features; high CSF protein; mitochondrial deletions on DNA testing |
| NADH–CoQ reductase deficiency | Pain, weakness, fatigue; worse with exercise | Exercise testing; confirmation by muscle biopsy |
| Cytochrome *b* deficiency | As in NADH–CoQ, plus mild weakness between attacks, ptosis in some cases | Exercise testing; confirmation by muscle biopsy |
| Cytochrome oxidase deficiency | As with cytochrome *b* deficiency | Exercise testing; confirmation by muscle biopsy |

PFK = phosphofructokinase; LDH = lactate dehydrogenase; CK = creatine kinase; EMG = electromyography; CPT = carnitine palmityltransferase; CSF = cerebrospinal fluid; NADH–CoQ = nicotinamide adenine dinucleotide–coenzyme Q.

autosomal dominant. Diagnosis is confirmed by the presence of low potassium levels during an attack. Provocative testing can be performed with an oral glucose load. Muscle biopsy may be normal or show some myopathic changes. NCVs are normal between attacks.

Hyperkalemic periodic paralysis presents with attacks of weakness but the potassium is usually elevated. This paralysis is also inherited as autosomal dominant. Normokalemic periodic paralysis has also been described. Hyper- and hypokalemic periodic paralyses can also be associated with other metabolic disorders, including thyrotoxicosis and renal failure, and with use of some drugs.

### Endocrine Myopathies

Hyperthyroidism is associated with multiple symptoms including tremor, irritability, heat intolerance, weight loss, and weakness. Neuromuscular disorders associated with thyrotoxicosis include myasthenia gravis, periodic paralysis, and myopathy.

Hypothyroidism is associated with lethargy, weakness, and cold intolerance. Neuromuscular findings may be proximal weakness and percussion myotonia, with associated delayed relaxation of tendon reflexes.

## NEUROMUSCULAR TRANSMISSION DEFECTS

Neuromuscular transmission defects present with weakness and fatigability. These defects are all due to impaired synaptic transmission, either from impaired ACh release from the presynaptic terminal or reduced available AChRs on the postsynaptic terminal. The essential features of the major neuromuscular transmission defects are shown in Table 5.12.

**Table 5.12   Neuromuscular Transmission Defects**

| Disorder | Clinical Features | Electrophysiologic Findings |
|----------|-------------------|-----------------------------|
| Myasthenia gravis | Weakness; worsens with activity | Normal CMAP; repetitive stimulation elicits decremental response with low stimulus rates; abnormal single-fiber EMG shows increased jitter and blocking |
| Myasthenic syndrome | Generalized or proximal weakness, often with dry mouth, impotence, and/or other autonomic signs | Decremental response at low rates; incremental at high rates; facilitation with exercise |
| Botulism | Prominent GI distress with abdominal cramping, diarrhea, and dry mouth, followed by generalized weakness with prominent bulbar involvement | Low CMAP amplitude, increases with exercise; repetitive stimulation elicits little or no decrement with low rates; incremental response seen with high rates |

CMAP = compound motor action potential; EMG = electromyography; GI = gastrointestinal.

## Myasthenia Gravis

Myasthenia gravis (MG) is an autoimmune disorder due to antibodies that bind to the AChRs, causing increased turnover; therefore, fewer receptors are available for binding with ACh. Most patients present with ocular motor weakness, characterized by diplopia and/or ptosis. The extraocular muscle weakness spans nerve distributions, which differentiates MG from single or multiple cranial nerve palsies. Patients with ocular MG have no axial or appendicular weakness, while patients with systemic MG present with proximal weakness that tends to be better in the morning.

NCVs are usually normal with single stimuli. EMG is usually normal. Repetitive stimulation of peripheral nerve at low rates (two to five stimulations per second) produces a decrement in the amplitude of the CMAP. Single-fiber EMG shows increased jitter and blocking, though these findings are not specific for MG and can be seen in denervating disorders.

## Botulism

Botulism is due to impaired release of ACh from the presynaptic terminal, resulting in less activation of the AChR. Patients present with autonomic symptoms, including abdominal cramps, diarrhea, and constipation, followed by generalized weakness including prominent ocular motor and bulbar involvement. Pupil constriction is impaired. CMAP amplitude is reduced. Repetitive stimulation at low rates (two to five stimulations per second) causes no decrement, but after exercise the amplitude of the response is increased. Repetitive stimulation at high rates (20 to 50 stimulations per second) reveals an incremental response to successive stimuli in the train. The response seen is often patchy, with some muscles being normal.

## Myasthenic (Eaton–Lambert) Syndrome

Myasthenic syndrome is an autoimmune disorder in which antibodies act at the presynaptic terminal to impair the release of ACh. Most patients with this syndrome have cancer, so it is usually a paraneoplastic disorder. Myasthenic syndrome is also associated with other autoimmune diseases, including systemic lupus erythematous and polymyositis.

Myasthenic syndrome presents with proximal or generalized weakness. Autonomic symptoms, including dry mouth and impotence, often develop, although they are less severe than those seen with botulism. Ophthalmoplegia or ptosis is unusual.

Motor NCV is normal but the CMAP is of low amplitude. Sensory NCV and SNAP amplitude are normal. Repetitive stimulation shows a decremental response at low rates of stimulation; after exercise, CMAP amplitude is markedly increased but the decremental response persists. High rates of stimulation produce an incremental response.

# Appendix

**Table A.1   Upper Extremity Muscle Action**

| Movement | Muscle(s) |
|---|---|
| Scapula elevation | Trapezius |
| Scapula adduction | Rhomboids |
| Scapula fixation against chest | Serratus anterior |
| Arm abduction | Deltoid, supraspinatus |
| Arm adduction | Teres major, latissimus dorsi |
| Arm internal rotation | Latissimus dorsi, teres major |
| Arm external rotation | Infraspinatus, teres minor |
| Forearm flexion | Biceps, brachialis, brachioradialis |
| Forearm extension | Triceps, anconeus |
| Forearm pronation | Pronator teres, pronator quadratus |
| Forearm supination | Supinator |
| Wrist flexion | Palmaris longus |
|   To radial side |     Flexor carpi radialis |
|   To ulnar side |     Flexor carpi ulnaris |
| Wrist extension | Extensor carpi radialis longus and brevis |
| Thumb flexion | Superficial head of the flexor pollicis brevis, flexor pollicis longus |
| Thumb extension | Extensor pollicis longus and brevis |
| Thumb opposition | Opponens pollicis |
| Thumb abduction | Abductor pollicis brevis and longus |
| Finger extension | Extensor digitorum, extensor indicis (index finger) |

**Table A.1** *(continued)*

| Movement | Muscle(s) |
|---|---|
| Finger flexion: digits 2 and 3 | Flexor digitorum profundus (median portion) |
| Finger flexion: digits 4 and 5 | Flexor digitorum profundus (ulnar portion) |
| Finger abduction | Interossei |
| Finger adduction | Lumbricals of hand |

**Table A.2 Upper Extremity Muscle Innervation**

| Muscle | Nerve | Plexus | Root |
|---|---|---|---|
| Abductor pollicis brevis | Median | CL, CM | C8–T1 |
| Abductor pollicis longus | Radial | CP | C7–8 |
| Anconeus | Radial | CP | C6–8 |
| Biceps | Musculocutaneous | CL | C5–6 |
| Brachialis | Musculocutaneous | CL | C5–7 |
| | Occasionally also radial | CP | C5–6 |
| Brachioradialis | Radial | CP | C5–6 |
| Deltoid | Axillary | CP | C5–6 |
| Extensor carpi radialis | | | |
| Longus | Radial | CP | C6–7 |
| Brevis | Posterior interosseus | CP | C6–7 |
| Extensor carpi ulnaris | Posterior interosseus | CP | C7–8 |
| Extensor digitorum | Posterior interosseus | CP | C7–8 |
| Extensor indicis | Posterior interosseus | CP | C7–8 |
| Extensor pollicis | | | |
| Longus | Posterior interosseus | CP | C7–8 |
| Brevis | Posterior interosseus | CP | C7–8 |
| Flexor carpi radialis | Median | CL, CM | C6–7 |
| Flexor carpi ulnaris | Ulnar | CM | C7–T1 |
| Flexor digitorum profundus | | | |
| Digits 2 and 3 | Anterior interosseus | CL, CM | C7–8 |
| Digits 4 and 5 | Ulnar | CM | C7–8 |
| Flexor digitorum super-ficialis | Median | CL, CM | C7–T1 |
| Flexor pollicis brevis | Median | CL, CM | C8–T1 |
| Infraspinatus | Suprascapular | TU | C5–6 |
| Interossei | Ulnar, deep branch | CM | C8–T1 |

**Table A.2** *(continued)*

| Muscle | Nerve | Plexus | Root |
|--------|-------|--------|------|
| Latisimus dorsi | Thoracodorsal | CP | C6–8 |
| Lumbricals | | | |
|    Digits 2 and 3 | Median | CL, CM | C8–T1 |
|    Digits 4 and 5 | Ulnar, deep branch | CM | C8–T1 |
| Opponens pollicis | Median | CL, CM | C8–T1 |
| Palmaris longus | Median | CL, CM | C7–T1 |
| Pronator quadratus | Anterior interosseus | CL, CM | C7–8 |
| Pronator teres | Median | CL, CM | C6–7 |
| | Occasionally musculo-cutaneous | CL | C5–7 |
| Rhomboids | Dorsal scapular | Direct from root | C5 |
| Serratus anterior | Long thoracic | Direct from roots | C5–7 |
| Supinator | Posterior interosseus | CP | C6–7 |
| Supraspinatus | Suprascapular | TU | C5–6 |
| Teres major | Subscapular | CP | C5–6 |
| Teres minor | Axillary | CP | C5–6 |
| Trapezius | Accessory nerve, with possible C3–4 contribution | — | — |
| Triceps | Radial | CP | C6–8 |

Note: Anterior interosseus is a branch of the median nerve, and posterior interosseus is a branch of the radial nerve.

CM = median cord, CL = lateral cord, CP = posterior cord; TU = upper trunk.

**Table A.3  Lower Extremity Muscle Action**

| *Movement* | *Muscle(s)* |
| --- | --- |
| Hip adduction | Adductor magnus, brevis, longus; obturator externus, pectineus |
| Hip abduction | Gluteus medius |
| Hip flexion | Iliopsoas, sartorius |
| Hip extension | Gluteus maximus |
| Hip eversion | Sartorius |
| Knee extension | Quadriceps |
| Knee flexion | Hamstrings (semimembranosus, semitendinosus) |
| Foot extension (dorsiflexion) | Tibialis anterior |
| Foot plantar flexion | Gastrocnemius, soleus, tibialis posterior, flexor digitorum longus, flexor hallucis longus |
| Foot inversion | Tibialis posterior |
| Foot eversion | Peroneus longus and brevis |
| Toe extension | Extensor hallucis longus |
| Great toe plantar flexion | Flexor hallucis longus |
| Toe plantar flexion (not including great toe) | Flexor digitorum longus |

**Table A.4   Lower Extremity Muscle Innervation**

| Muscle | Nerve | Plexus | Root |
|---|---|---|---|
| Adductor magnus | Obturator–posterior division | Lumbar | L2–4 |
| Biceps femoris | Sciatic | Sacral | L4–S2 |
| Extensor digitorum brevis | Deep peroneal | Sacral | L5–S1 |
| Extensor digitorum longus | Deep peroneal | Sacral | L5–S1 |
| Extensor hallucis longus | Deep peroneal | Sacral | L5–S1 |
| Flexor digitorum longus | Tibial | Sacral | L5–S2 |
| Flexor hallucis longus | Tibial | Sacral | S1–2 |
| Gastrocnemius | Tibial | Sacral | S1–2 |
| Gluteus maximus | Inferior gluteal | Sacral | L5–S2 |
| Gluteus medius | Superior gluteal | Sacral | L4–S1 |
| Iliopsoas | Lumbar plexus, branches of the femoral nerve | Lumbar | L2–4 |
| Peroneus longus, brevis, and tertius | Superficial peroneal | Sacral | L5–S1 |
| Quadriceps, including rectus femoris, vastus medialis, lateralis, and intermedius | Femoral | Lumbar | L2–4 |
| Sartorius | Femoral | Lumbar | L2–4 |
| Semimembranosus | Sciatic | Sacral | L4–S2 |
| Semitendinosus | Sciatic | Sacral | L4–S2 |
| Soleus | Tibial | Sacral | S1–2 |
| Tibialis anterior | Deep peroneal | Sacral | L4–5 |
| Tibialis posterior | Tibial | Sacral | L4–5 |

## Table A.5 Axonal Neuropathies

**Acute and Subacute**

Diabetic amyotrophy

Mononeuropathy multiplex; individual nerves present acutely

Nutritionally based, due to $B_{12}$ deficiency, alcoholism

Toxic, due to vincristine, cisplatin, hydralazine, triorithocresylphosphate (TOCP)

Vasculitis

**Chronic**

Diabetic sensorimotor neuropathy

Metabolic, due to uremia, storage diseases

Hereditary neuropathies

    Hereditary motor–sensory neuropathy (HMSN) II (neuronal Charcot–Marie–Tooth disease)

    Hereditary sensory neuropathies

Amyloid neuropathy

Toxic (as above)

## Table A.6 Demyelinating Neuropathies

**Acute and Subacute**

Guillain–Barré syndrome (or acute inflammatory demyelinating polyradiculoneuropathy)

**Chronic**

Chronic inflammatory demyelinating polyradiculoneuropathy

Hereditary motor–sensory neuropathy (HMSN) I (hypertrophic Charcot–Marie–Tooth disease)

HMSN III (Dejerine–Sottas disease)

**Table A.7   Neuronopathies**

**Pure Motor**

Upper and lower motoneuron

Amyotrophic lateral sclerosis (ALS)

Familial ALS

Lower motoneuron only

Spinal muscular atrophy

Type 1: infantile (Werdnig–Hoffman disease)

Type 2: late infantile

Type 3: juvenile (Kugelberg–Welander disease)

Type 4: adult

Poliomyelitis

Upper motoneuron only

Primary lateral sclerosis

**Pure Sensory**

Paraneoplastic sensory neuropathy

Friedreich's ataxia, early in course

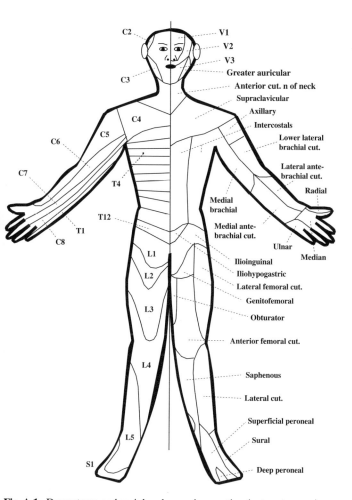

**Fig. A.1** Dermatome and peripheral nerve innervation (cut., cutaneous).

# Index

Abdominal reflexes, 151
Abducens nerve (CN VI), 72, 80, 83, 84, 109, 130, 131, 149
  palsy, 14, 80, 83, 84, 90, 108, 111, 168
Abscess, cerebral, 22
Accessory nerve (CN XI), 72, 103, 105–106, 118–120
  palsy, 149
Acetylcholine, 155
Achilles tendon reflex, 153, 177
Acid maltase deficiency, 186
Acoustic nerve, 1
Acoustic neuroma, 101
Acute encephalitis, 16–17
Acute inflammatory demyelinating polyradiculoneuropathy, 169
Acute neuropathies, 165
Adie's syndrome, 93
Affect, cerebral anatomy, 4–6
Afferent pupil, 91–92
Akinesia, 24, 38
Akinetic mutism, 19, 28
Akinetic rigid syndromes
  diffuse Lewy body disease, 43, 44, 56
  drug-induced parkinsonism, 55–56
  multiple system atrophy, 55, 131
  olivopontecerebellar atrophy, 55, 59, 126, 131

Parkinson's disease, 45, 54–56, 59, 132
  progressive supranuclear palsy, 46, 55, 56–57, 59
  Shy–Drager syndrome, 55, 131
  striatonigral degeneration, 55, 56
Alcoholic cerebellar degeneration, 124
Alertness, 66
Alexia, 31, 39, 49
Alzheimer's disease, 8, 43–44
Amino acid defects, 59
Amyloidosis, 93
Amyotrophic lateral sclerosis (ALS), 141, 164
  differential diagnosis, 146, 150–151, 163, 164, 167, 181
  spinal cord, 141
Angular gyrus, 2, 30–31
Aniscoria, 92
Ankle tendon reflex, 142
Anomia, 31, 39, 41
Anosmia, 73, 129
Anoxic encephalopathy, 8–10
Anterior cerebral artery, 24–25, 34, 36
Anterior cingulate gyrus, 19
Anterior inferior cerebellar artery (AICA), 123
Anterior interosseus syndrome, 175
Anterior spinal artery, 138

Anterior spinal artery syndrome, 139, 141, 147–148, 151
Anterolateral tract, 134, 135, 137
Antiphospholipid antibody syndrome, 22
Anton's syndrome, 48
Aphasia, 42
  Alzheimer's disease, 43–44
  anomia, 31, 39, 41
  Broca's a (anterior) a., 25, 39, 40
  conduction a., 31, 37, 40, 42
  global a., 40, 41
  transcortical a., 39–42, 68–69
  Wernicke's (posterior) a., 25, 39–41
Aphemia, 39
Apraxia, 24, 49, 50
  constructional apraxia, 38, 59
  ideational apraxia, 35
  ideomotor apraxia, 31, 36–37
  limb-kinetic apraxia, 35
  for objects, 35, 37
  oculomotor apraxia, 93
  parietal lobe lesions, 31
  for sequential tasks, 35, 37
Aqueduct obstruction, 15
Arbovirus encephalitis, 17–18
Arcuate fasciculus, 3, 37
Areflexia, 159
Argyll Robertson pupil, 92, 93, 143
Arnold–Chiari malformation, 127–128, 144
Arteries *see* individual arteries
Artery of Adamkiewicz, 138, 147
Ataxia, 125–126
  autosomal dominant cerebellar ataxia, 126–127
  cerebellar ataxia, 66, 115, 121, 123–126

Friedreich's ataxia, 125
frontal lobe ataxia, 28
idiopathic progressive ataxia, 126
paraneoplastic cerebellar degeneration, 127
peri-infectious cerebellar dysfunction, 127
Ramsay Hunt syndrome, 98–99, 125–126
slowly progressive ataxia, 121–122
viral infection, 127
Ataxia telangiectasia, 59
Ataxic hemiparesis, 108
Athetoid cerebral palsy, 63
Athetosis, 58, 59, 60
Autoimmune myopathies, 182–183
Autonomic neuropathies, 165
Autosomal dominant cerebellar ataxia (ADCA), 126–127
Axonal neuropathy, 165, 167, 168, 197
Axonopathy, 160
Axonotmesis, 165

Back pain, spinal lesions, 139–153
Bacterial myositis, 185
Ballism, 58, 59
Basal ganglia, 51–53, 63
  calcification, 60
  hemorrhage, 26
Basal ganglia dysfunction, 12–13, 60
Basal ganglia lesions, 54, 60
  akinetic rigid syndromes, 54–57
  dystonia and dyskinesia, 58–67
  tremor, 57–58
Basal ganglia loop, 66

Basilar artery, 112, 114, 116
    infarction, 117, 130
    thrombosis, 114, 130–131
    top-of-the-basilar syndrome, 68,
        108, 114, 132
Behavior, cerebral anatomy, 4–6,
    28, 32
Bell's palsy, 98
Benign intracranial hypertension,
    14
Benign positional vertigo, 101
Biceps reflex, 150
Blepharospasm, 61
Blink reflex, 29
Botulism, 188, 189
Brachial plexitis, 173, 178
Brachial plexopathy, 173
Brachial plexus, 173–174
Brain abscess, 22
Brain stem, 53, 107–110
    degeneration, 56
    destruction, 19
    encephalitis, 93
    eye movement control, 75,
        77–79
    inputs, 138
    medulla, 118–121
    midbrain, 78–79, 109, 112–115
    outputs, 51, 66, 121
    views, 73, 110, 113, 115, 120,
        122
Brain stem lesions, 108, 110–112,
    149
    different from vestibulocochlear
        lesion, 100–101
    eye movements, 85
    facial weakness, 97, 98
Brancher glycogen storage
    disease, 186
Broca's aphasia, 25, 40

Broca's area, 2, 25
Brown–Séquard syndrome, 139,
    141, 142–143
Bulbospinal tracts, 133–137
Butterfly gliomas, 30

Cancer, 20, 22–23, 185; *see also*
    Tumors
Carbon monoxide poisoning, 60
Carnitine palmityl transference
    (CPT) deficiency, 186
Carpal tunnel syndrome, 164, 175
Cauda equina syndrome, 139, 153
Caudate nucleus, 51, 53, 62
Cavernous sinus, 89
Cavernous sinus syndrome, 129
Central cord lesions, 86
Central cord syndrome, 139, 150
Central nystagmus, 87
Central pontine myelinolysis, 88
Central reflex pathways, 156
Cerebellar ataxia, 66, 115, 121,
    123–126
Cerebellar dysfunction, 121–127
Cerebellar hemorrhage, 27, 124
Cerebellar infarctions, 123
Cerebellar loop, 66
Cerebellar peduncles, 121
Cerebellar stroke, 123
Cerebellar tonsils, 127
Cerebellar tremor, 57
Cerebellar tumors, 124
Cerebellopontine angle syndrome,
    129–130
Cerebellum, 53, 120–128
Cerebral cortex and white matter,
    53, 66
    akinesia, 24, 38
    anatomy, 1–33
    aphasia, 25, 31, 39–42, 68–69

Cerebral cortex and white matter
(*Cont.*):
  apraxia, 35–38, 49, 50, 59, 93
  arteries, 24–26
  dementia, 42–46
  facial weakness, 97
  functions, 1–7
  lesions *see* Cerebral lesions
  localization
    functional, 1–7
    pathologic, 8–33
  motor and sensory dysfunction,
    33–42
  sensory loss, 34–35
  visual field abnormalities,
    46–49
  visuospatial dysfunction, 49–50
  weakness, 33
Cerebral hemispheres, views, 2, 3,
  5, 24
Cerebral lesions
  cortical l., 8, 31
  diffuse cerebral l., 8–20
  eye movement, 82
  facial weakness, 97
  focal cerebral l., 23–33
  hypothalamic l., 4
  left hemisphere l., 4, 41, 49, 50
  multifocal cerebral l., 20–23
  posterior fossa l., 14, 16
  right hemisphere l., 4, 49, 50
  subcortical l., 8
  temporal lobe l., 4
Cerebral lobular hemorrhage, 26
Cerebral palsy (CP), 12–13, 63
Cerebral peduncles, 112
Cerebral vascular infarction,
  25–26, 30, 33, 40
Cerebral vascular lesions, sensory
  loss, 36

Cerebral vascular syndromes, 23,
  25–27
Cervical cord lesions, 150–151
Cervical radiculopathy, 172
Cervical spondylosis, 150–151
Cervical sympathetic chain, 86
Cervical syrinx, 144
Cervicomedullary junction, 88
Charcot joints, 143
Charcot–Marie–Tooth (CMT)
  disease, 170–171
Chorda tympani, 96
Chorea, 58–59, 60
Chorea gravidarum, 60
Choreoathetosis, 60, 62, 64
Claustrum, 51
Clumsy hand–dysarthria
  syndrome, 108, 118–119
CNS vasculitis, 21–22
Cochlea, 99
Communicating hydrocephalus, 15
Complex partial seizures, 5–6
Compound motor action potential
  (CMAP), 160–161, 164
Conduction block neuropathy, 164
Constructional apraxia, 38, 59
Conus medullaris, 153
Convergence–retraction
  nystagmus, 114
Copper metabolism, Wilson's
  disease, 63
Cori's disease, 186
Corrective eye movements, 75, 76
Cortical blindness, 48, 132
Cortical lesions, 8, 31
Cortical sensory loss, 31, 34, 35
Cortical visual areas, 47
Corticospinal tract, 111, 115, 118,
  119, 132, 134–138

Corticospinal tract signs, 140
Cranial nerve palsy, 14, 17
  CN III (ocular motor nerve), 14,
      80, 83, 89–90, 108, 114,
      168
  CN IV (trochlear nerve), 14, 83,
      90, 114
  CN VI (abducens palsy), 14, 80,
      83, 84, 90, 108, 111, 168
  CN VII (facial nerve), 84, 108,
      109
  CN IX to XII, 149
  single/multiple, 111
  spinal cord lesions, 149
Cranial nerves, table, 72; *see also*
      Cranial nerve palsy;
      individual nerves
Craniocervical junction lesions,
      149
Creatine kinase (CK) level, 162
Cytochrome *b* deficiency, 187
Cytochrome oxidase deficiency,
      187

Dandy–Walker syndrome, 129
Debrancher deficiency, 186
Deep tendon reflexes (DTRs),
      165, 166
Defective neuronal migration,
      18–19
Dejerine–Sottas disease, 109, 171
Dementia, 42–46
  Alzheimer's disease, 43–44
  apraxia, 37
  cortrical dementias, 42, 43–44
  diffuse Lewy body disease, 43,
      44, 56
  Huntington's disease, 43
  hydrocephalus, 15
  multi-infarct dementia, 45

multiple sclerosis, 45
Parkinson's disease, 45, 54
Pick's disease, 44
progressive supranuclear palsy,
      46, 57
subcortical dementias, 43, 45–46
thalamic degeneration, 68
vascular dementia, 45
Demyelinating neuropathy, 160,
      164, 167, 169, 170–171,
      197
Depression, 4
Dermatomyositis, 161, 182–184,
      185
Developmental disorders, 18–20
Diabetic neuropathy, 164, 168–169
Diabetic polyradiculopathy, 169
Diffuse cerebral edema, 13
Diffuse cerebral lesions, 8–20
  apraxia, 37
  cerebral palsy, 12–13
  encephalopathy, anoxic, 8–12
  hydrocephalus, 14–16
  increased intracranial pressure,
      13–16
Diffuse Lewy body disease, 43,
      44, 56
Diplegia, watershed infarcts, 13
Diplopia, aqueduct obstruction, 15
Dopa-responsive dystonia, 61
Dorsal columns, 134, 135, 137
Dorsal funiculus, 137
Dorsal roots, tabes dorsalis, 143
Downbeat nystagmus, 84, 88, 149
Drug exposure
  chorea, 60
  dystonia, 59
  encephalopathy, 12
  oculogyric crisis, 88–89
  parkinsonism, 55–56

Drug exposure (*Cont.*):
   recurrent laryngeal nerve palsy,
     105
   tardive dyskinesia, 65
   tremor, 58
Duchenne muscular dystrophy,
    162, 183
Dysarthria, 108, 118–119
Dysesthesia, 164
Dyskinesia, 58–59
   athetoid cerebral palsy, 63
   Hallervorden–Spatz disease, 59,
    60, 64
   hemiballismus, 65
   hemifacial spasm, 65, 99
   Huntington's disease, 62–63
   kernicterus, 64
   paroxysmal choreoathetosis, 62,
    64
   Sydenham's chorea, 63
   tardive dyskinesia, 65
   Wilson's disease, 63
Dysphonia, 62
Dystonia, 58, 59, 61, 62

Eaton–Lambert syndrome, 188,
    189
Edinger–Westphal nucleus, 74, 78
Electrocerebral silence (ECS), 10
Electroencephalography (EEG),
    anoxia, 10
Electromyography (EMG),
    159–161, 162
Emery–Dreifuss muscular
    dystrophy, 183
Encephalitis, 16–18, 93
Encephalopathy, 8–12
Endocrine myopathy, 187–188
Enhanced physiologic tremor, 57,
    58

Epidural hematoma, 23, 148
Essential tremor, 57–58
Evoked potentials, 21
Extramedullary tumors, 141–142
Extraocular muscles, 90–91, 155
Eye movements, 9–10; *see also*
    Ocular motor dysfunction;
    Ocular motor nerve;
    Ocular motor system;
    Optic nerve
   abnormalities, 133
   control, 76–80
   encephalopathy, 9–10
   examination, 80–82
   ocular bobbing, 84, 88
   pontine gaze center, 77–78
   types, 75–76
Eyes; *see also* Ocular motor
    nerve; Ocular motor
    system; Optic nerve
   blepharospasm, 61
   eyelid elevation, 79
   proptosis, 75, 130
   pupil diameter, 74, 78
   pupillary abnormalities, 68, 89,
    91–93, 114, 132, 143
   Wilson's disease diagnosis, 63

Face, innervation, 35
Facial canal, 97
Facial nerve (CN VII), 72, 79, 80,
    84, 95–99, 109, 117, 119,
    123, 149
   palsy, 84, 108, 109
Facial weakness, 96–97
Facioscapulohumeral muscular
    dystrophy, 183
Familial dysautonomia, 172
Familial hypokalemic periodic
    paralysis, 184

Femoral neuropathy, 180
Flocculonodular lobe, 121
Focal cerebral lesions
    apraxia, 37
    frontal lobe l., 23–30
    occipital lobe l., 33
    parasagittal l., 33
    parietal lobe l., 30–31
    temporal lobe l., 32
Focal dystonias, 61–62
Focal infarcts, cerebral palsy, 13
Focal seizures, 17
Foix–Alajouanine syndrome, 148
Foster Kennedy syndrome, 128
Foville's syndrome, 109, 117
Friedreich's ataxia, 126
Frontal lobe lesions, 23–30
    akinesia, 38
    apraxia, 37
    ataxia, 28
    eye movement, 82–83
    gaze abnormalities, 77
    infarctions, 25, 30

Gag reflexes, 103
Gait abnormalities, 124, 149
Gaze abnormalities, 77–78, 83, 84,
        87, 132
    internuclear ophthalmoplegia,
        77–78, 84, 86
    one-and-a-half syndrome, 86–87
Generalized neuropathies, 167
Geniculate ganglion, 96, 97
Genioglossus muscles, 106–107
Geniohyoid muscles, 106–107
Gerstmann's syndrome, 31
Glabellar reflex, 29
Glaucoma, 93
Gliomas, 30, 75, 129
Globus pallidus, 46, 51–53, 64, 66

Glomus jugulare tumors, 103
Glossopharyngeal nerve (CN IX),
        72, 102–103, 110, 120
    palsy, 149
Glossopharyngeal neuralgia, 103
Glycogen storage disorders, 161,
        186
Gradenigo's syndrome, 80, 130
Grasp reflex, 29
Gray matter, 132, 140
Guillain–Barre syndrome, 163,
        164, 169–170
Gunn pupil, 91–92

Hallervorden–Spatz disease, 59,
        60, 64
Hallucinations, 49
Hand, innervation, 35
Head injury, 23, 30, 32, 73
Hearing, 1, 99–100
Hematomas, 23, 148
Hemianopia, 31, 47
Hemiballismus, 59, 65
Hemifacial spasm, 65, 99
Hemiparesis, 108, 117–118
Hemorrhage
    basal ganglia h., 26
    cerebellar h., 27, 124
    cerebral lobe h., 26
    epidural h., 23, 27
    intraparenchymal h., 148–149
    parenchymal h., 13
    periventricular h., 13
    pons h., 27
    spinal cord lesions, 148–149
    subarachnoid h., 13–14, 15, 148
    subdural h., 23, 27
Hereditary motor–sensory
        neuropathy (HMSN),
        170–171

Hereditary neuropathies, 170–172
Hereditary sensory neuropathy,
171–172
Herpes simplex, 17
Herpes zoster, 80, 95, 98–99
Heschl's gyrus, 1, 32
Hippocampus, 32
Hippus, 92
Holoprosencephaly, 18
Horner's syndrome, 84, 85–86, 92,
124
Humeroperoneal muscular
dystrophy, 183
Huntington's disease, 54, 59, 60,
62–63
dementia, 43
Hydrocephalus, 13, 14–16
akinetic mutism, 19
aqueductal obstruction, 15
communicating, h., 15
Dandy–Walker syndrome, 129
mass lesions, 16
normal pressure h., 15
obstructive h., 14, 125
Parinaud's syndrome, 114
unilateral h., 16
Hydromyelia, 144
Hyperreflexia, 181
Hypertension, intracranial, 14
Hyperthyroidism, 187
Hypoglossal nerve (CN XII), 72,
103, 106–107, 110
palsy, 149
Hyporeflexia, 159
Hypothalamic lesions, 4
Hypothyroidism, 188

Immediate recall, 6
Immunoglobulin G, multiple
sclerosis, 20–21

Inclusion body myositis, 185
Incongruous field defect, 47
Infarctions
anterior spinal artery syndrome,
147–148
basilar i., 117, 131
cerebellar i., 124
cerebral vascular i., 25–26, 30,
33, 40
focal i., 13
frontal lobe i., 25, 30
lacunar i., 117
medullary i., 121, 123
midbrain i., 123
multiple i., 21–22, 45
occipital i., 48
paramedian brain stem i., 78
Parinaud's syndrome, 114
PICA i., 120, 123
posterior spinal artery
occlusion, 148
skew deviation, 87
thalamic i., 42
watershed i., 13, 42
Inferior colliculus, 66
Inferior parietal lobule, 2, 30
Inflammatory myopathy, 161, 162,
185
Internal auditory canal, 96, 97
Internal capsule, 34, 97
Internuclear ophthalmoplegia
(INO), 77–78, 84, 86, 111
Intradural tumors, 141, 142
Intramedullary tumors, 141, 142
Ipsilateral eye fibers, 67
Ischemia, 89

Junctional scotoma, 47, 75

Kayser–Fleischer ring, 63

Kearns–Sayre syndrome, 187
Kernicterus, 63
Kugelberg–Welander disease, 146

Lacunar infarction, 118
Language, 1–3, 6, 31
Language disorders *see* Aphasia
Lateral femoral cutaneous
        neuropathy, 180
Lateral gaze palsy, 77
Lateral geniculate body, 46, 48,
        67, 74
Lateral medullary syndrome, 109,
        120, 123
Lateral rectus palsy, 130
Lateral spinothalamic tract, 134
LDH deficiency, 186
Learning, 6–7
Left cerebral hemisphere, views,
        2, 5, 24, 52
Left frontal lobe, focal lesions, 83
Left gaze preference, 84
Left hemisphere lesions, 4, 41, 49,
        50
Legs
    dystonia, 61
    spinal lesions, 138–153
    spinal stenosis, 152
    vascular claudication, 152
    weakness, 34, 140, 159
Leigh disease, 59
Lenticulostriate artery, 36
Lentiform nucleus, 51
Leprosy, 162
Lesch–Nyhan syndrome, 59
Ligament of Struthers syndrome,
        175
Limb-girdle muscular dystrophy,
        183
Limbic system, function, 5, 6–7

Limb-kinetic apraxia, 35–36
Lipid storage disorders, 161, 186
Lissencephaly, 18
Locked-in syndrome, 9, 19–20,
        108, 117, 131, 149
Long-term memory, 6, 7
Lumbar cord lesions, 151–153
Lumbar plexitis, 178
Lumbar spondylosis, 151–152
Lumbosacral plexopathy, 177–178
Lumbosacral plexus, 178
Lumbosacral radiculopathy, 177
Lymphomas, 142

Man-in-a-barrel syndrome, 150
Mastoid infection, 80
McArdle's disease, 186
Medial geniculate body, 66
Medial lemniscus, 112, 115
Medial longitudinal fasciculus
        (MLF), 77, 83, 86, 111,
        112, 115, 134
Medial medullary syndrome, 109,
        120
Medial rectus muscle, 91
Medial temporal lobe, 32
Median neuropathy, 173, 175
Medular lesions, 109, 120
Medulla, 118–121
Medullary infarction, 120, 124
Meige syndrome, 62
Memory, cerebral anatomy, 6–7
Memory disorders, 32, 68
Meniere's disease, 102
Meningiomas, 29, 30, 75,
        124–125, 129
Meningitis, neoplastic, 139
Metabolic encephalopathy, 10–12
Metabolic myopathy, 184, 186–187
Metachromatic leukodystrophy, 59

Meyer's loop, 32
Microcephaly, 18
Midbrain, 78–79, 109, 112–115
Midbrain infarction, 123
Midbrain lesions, 83, 114
Middle cerebral artery, 24–26, 33, 36, 40, 41
Millard–Gubler syndrome, 83, 84, 108, 117
Mitochondrial myopathy, 161, 187
Mononeuron disease, 181–182
Mononeuropathy, 165, 172–181
   brachial plexopathy, 173
   cervical radiculopathy, 172
   femoral neuropathy, 180
   lateral femoral cutaneous neuropathy, 180
   lumbosacral plexopathy, 177–178
   lumbosacral radiculopathy, 177
   median neuropathy, 173, 175
   obturator neuropathy, 180–181
   peroneal neuropathy, 179
   radial neuropathy, 175, 176
   sciatic neuropathy, 179
   tarsal tunnel syndrome, 180
   tibial neuropathy, 179–180
   ulnar neuropathy, 173, 176
Mononeuropathy multiplex, 168, 181
Motor dysfunction, 33–38, 54–65, 69
Motor function, 4, 51, 53, 121, 138, 137
Motor neurons, 155
Motor neuropathy, 160, 163–164, 182
Multifocal cerebral lesions, 20–23
Multifocal motor neuropathy, 182
Multifocal neuropathy, 159, 167

Multi-infarct dementia (MID), 45
Multiple sclerosis (MS), 8, 20–21
   dementia, 45
   dizziness, 102
   eye movements, 78, 87
   optic neuritis, 20, 75
   spinal cord, 144
Multiple system atrophy, 55, 131
Muscle biopsy, 161
Muscle fiber membrane, 155
Muscle phosphrylase deficiency, 186
Muscles; *see also* individual muscles; Myopathy
   action, 155, 157
   lower extremity, 195–196
   strength scale, 157
   upper extremity, 191–194
Muscular dystrophy, 161, 162, 183
Myasthenia gravis, 91, 187, 188, 189
Myasthenic syndrome, 161, 189
Myelitis, 20, 143–144
Myelopathy, parasagittal lesions, 33
Myopathy, 160, 182–188
   diagnosis, 161
   endocrine myopathies, 187–188
   metabolic myopathies, 184, 186–187
   muscular dystrophies, 182, 183
   periodic paralysis, 184, 187
Myositis, 185
Myotonic muscular dystrophy, 183

NADH-CoQ reductase deficiency, 187
Nasociliary nerve, 79
Nasopharyngeal lesions, 103

Neglect (visuospatial dysfunction), 50, 68
Neoplastic meningitis, 139
Nerve biopsy, 161–162
Nerve conduction velocity (NCV), 159–161, 163–164
Nerves; *see also* individual nerves; Neuropathy; Plexopathy; Radiculopathy
  brachial plexus, 174
  chart, 174, 178, 199
  lower extremity, 196
  lumbosacral plexus, 178
  upper extremity, 193–194
Nervous tremor, 58
Nervus intermedius, 96
Neuralgia, 95, 103
Neurapraxia, 165
Neuroblastoma, 127
Neuromas, 130
Neuromuscular axis, 155–159
Neuromuscular disorders, differential diagnosis, 158–163
Neuromuscular junction, 155, 156, 159
Neuromuscular transmission defects, 160, 161, 178–179
Neuronal necrosis, cerebral palsy, 12
Neuronopathies, 166, 198
Neuropathy, 22, 158
  age of onset, 167
  axonal neuropathy, 165, 167, 168, 197
  chronicity, 163, 164
  demyelinating neuropathies, 160, 164, 167, 169, 170–171, 197
  differential diagnosis, 159–161, 162–167
  distribution, 164, 166–167
  modality, 163–165
  mononeuron disease, 181–182
  mononeuropathy, 172–181
  mononeuropathy multiplex, 168, 181
  pathology, 164, 165–166
  polyneuropathy, 167–172
Neurosyphilis, 143
Neurotmesis, 165
Niemann–Pick disease, 59
Normal pressure hydrocephalus, 15
Nucleus ambiguus, 118, 119
Nucleus cuneatus, 118, 119
Nucleus gracilis, 118, 119
Nucleus of the solitary tract, 96
Nystagmus, 81
  Arnold–Chiari malformation, 129
  central nystagmus, 87
  convergence–retraction nystagmus, 114
  downbeat nystagmus, 84, 88, 149
  horizontal nystagmus, 84, 87
  optokinetic nystagmus, 81–82
  peripheral nystagmus, 87
  vertical nystagmus, 84

Obstructive hydrocephalus, 14, 125
Obturator neuropathy, 180–181
Occipital lobe lesions, 33, 48, 49, 85
Ocular bobbing, 84, 88
Ocular motor dysfunction, 56, 62; *see also* Eye movements
Ocular motor apraxia, 93
Ocular motor system, 75–93

Oculogyric crisis, 88–89
Oculomotor nerve (CN III), 72,
  79–80, 83, 129, 130
  palsy, 14, 80, 89–90, 93, 108,
    114, 168
Oculomotor nuclear complex, 112
Oculopharyngeal muscular
  dystrophy, 183
Olfactory groove tumors, 29, 74
Olfactory nerve (CN I), 71–74
Olfactory nerve lesions, 73
Oligodendrogliomas, 126
Olivopontocerebellar atrophy
  (OPA), 55, 59, 126, 131
One-and-a-half syndrome, 86–87,
  111
Optic canal, 74
Optic chiasm, 46, 48, 67, 74
Optic nerve (CN II), 14, 46, 48,
  67, 71, 74–75, 109
Optic nerve lesions, 74–75
Optic neuritis, 20, 75
Optic radiations, 46–47, 48, 67
Optic tracts, 46, 48, 67, 109
Optokinetic nystagmus (OKN),
  81–82
Oromandibular dystonia, 61–62

Pachygyria, 18
Palatal reflexes, 103
Palmomental reflex, 29
Palsy
  abducens p., 14, 80, 83, 84, 90,
    108, 111
  athetoid cerebral p., 63
  Bell's p., 98
  cerebral p., 12–13
  cranial nerve p. *see* Cranial
    nerve palsy
  lateral gaze p., 77

  lateral rectus p., 130
  ocular motor p., 14
  peroneal nerve p., 179
  progressive supranuclear p., 46,
    56
  pseudobulbar p., 105
  recurrent laryngeal nerve p.,
    105
  Saturday night p., 175
Paramedian brain stem infarction,
  78
Paramedian pontine reticular
  formation (PPRF), 76, 77,
  86, 115
Paraneoplastic cerebellar
  degeneration, 127
Parasagittal lesions, 30, 33, 138
Parasitic myositis, 185
Paratonia, 27, 38, 54
Parenchymal hematoma, 23
Paresthesia, 164
Parietal lobe lesions, 30–31, 85
Parinaud's syndrome, 83, 84
Parkinsonism, 24, 27, 28, 38
  different from essential tremor,
    58
  drug-induced, 55–56
Parkinson's disease (PD), 54–56,
  59
  dementia, 45, 54
  Shy–Drager syndrome different
    from, 131
  tremor, 55, 57, 58
Paroxysmal choreoathetosis, 60,
  64
Patellar reflex, 177, 180
Patellar tendon, 177
Periodic paralysis
  Hyperkalemic, 187
  Hypokalemic, 184

Peripheral nerves, 34, 155–157, 199
Peripheral nystagmus, 87
Peripheral vestibulopathy, 101–102
Periventricular hemorrhage, 13
Peroneal neuropathy, 179
Persistent vegetative state, 19
Phosphofrucyokinase (PFK) deficiency, 186
Phosphoglycerate kinase deficiency, 186
Pick's disease, 44
Pinealomas, 93
Pituitary tumors, 75
Plexitis, 173, 178
Plexopathy, 173, 177–178
Plexus, sensory loss, 34
Poliomyelitis, 182
Polymyalgia rheumatica, 185
Polymyositis, 161, 182–184, 185
Polyneuropathy, 167–172
   CIDP, 164, 170
   diabetic neuropathy, 168–169
   Guillain–Barré syndrome, 163, 164, 169–170
   hereditary neuropathies, 170–172
Polyradiculoneuropathy, 164, 169, 170
Polyradiculopathy, diabetic, 169
Pompe's disease, 186
Pons, 27, 97, 109
Pontine gaze center, 77–78
Pontine lesions, 108–109, 116–119
   facial weakness, 97
   gaze abnormalities, 77, 83, 88
Pontomedullary junction, 116
Postcentral gyrus, 4, 30, 66
Posterior aphasia, 39, 40–41
Posterior auricular nerve, 96

Posterior cerebral artery, 24, 25, 48, 67
Posterior fossa, 16, 125
Posterior inferior cerebellar artery (PICA), 120, 123
Posterior nuclear group, 66
Posterior spinal arteries, 138, 148
Precentral gyrus, 4, 33, 66, 135
Pregnancy, chorea, 60
Premotor area, 4, 37, 38, 66
Primary auditory cortex, 6, 32, 100
Primary visual cortex, 3–4, 74
Progressive muscular atrophy (PMA), 147
Progressive supranuclear palsy, 46, 55, 56–57, 59
Pronator teres syndrome, 175
Proptosis, 75, 129
Pseudobulbar palsy, 105
Pseudotumor cerebri, 14
Pupil diameter, 74, 78
Pupillary abnormalities, 68, 89, 91–93, 114, 132, 143
Pure motor hemiparesis, 117, 118
Pure word deafness, 32
Purkinje cells, 128
Pursuit eye movements, 75, 76
Putamen, 51, 53

Quadriparesis, 150

Radial neuropathy, 175, 176
Radiation plexopathy, 173
Radiculopathy
   cervical radiculopathy, 172
   diabetic polyradiculopathy, 169
   lumboscaral, 177
   spondylosis, 150
Raeder's paratrigeminal neuralgia, 95

Rage, 4–5
Ramsay Hunt syndrome, 98–99, 126
Reading, 2, 31, 32
    *see also* Alexia
Recurrent laryngeal nerve, 104, 105
Red nucleus, 112, 123
Reflexes, 29, 103, 150, 151, 153, 158, 159, 165, 177
    abdominal r., 151
    Achilles tendon r., 153, 177
    ankle tendon r., 153
    areflexia, 159
    biceps r., 150
    blink r., 29
    central reflex pathways, 156
    deep tendon r., 165, 166
    gag r., 103
    glabellar r., 29
    grading scale, 158
    grasp r., 29
    hyperreflexia, 181
    hyporeflexia, 159
    palatal r., 103
    palmomental r., 29
    patellar r., 177, 180
    plantar r., 158
    rooting r., 29
    snout r., 29
    suck r., 29
Refsum disease, 171
Reticulospinal tract, 134
Retinal lesions, 92
Retinal nerves, 74
Rheumatic fever, Sydenham's chorea, 673
Right cerebral hemisphere, 3, 4, 49, 50
Right superior quadrant defect, 47

Riley–Day syndrome, 172
Rooting reflex, 29
Rubrospinal tract, 134, 138–137

Saccadic eye movements, 75–77
Sacral cord lesions, 153
Sarcoidosis, 93
Saturday night palsy, 175
Scapuloperoneal muscular dystrophy, 183
Schwann cells, 155
Schwannoma, 101
Sciatic neuropathy, 179
Seizures, 5–6, 12, 17, 62
Sensorimotor neuropathy, 164, 168
Sensory dysfunction, 33–38, 68
Sensory function, cerebral anatomy, 4, 30
Sensory nerve action potential (SNAP), 160–161
Sensory neuronopathy, 160
Sensory neuropathy, 164, 168–169
Sensory strip, 30, 35
Shy–Drager syndrome, 55, 131
Skew deviation, 84, 87
Smell, 71–74
Solitary tract nucleus, 120
Somatosensory cortex, 4
Somatosensory system, 4, 66
Spasmodic dysphonia, 62
Spasmodic torticollis, 61
Speech, 2, 30–31; *see also* Aphasia
Spinal arteries, 138
Spinal cord, 53
    anatomy, 133–138
    sensory loss, 34
    tracts, 133–135
    tumors affecting, 141
    views, 134

Spinal cord lesions, 138–153
  amyotrophic lateral sclerosis,
    141, 146, 150–151, 163,
    164, 167, 181
  cauda equina syndrome, 139,
    153
  cervical cord, 150
  conus medullaris, 153
  craniocervical junction, 149
  hemorrhage, 148–149
  infarctions, 147–148
  localization, 138–140
  lumbar cord, 151–153
  multiple sclerosis, 144
  progressive muscular atrophy,
    147
  sacral cord, 153
  spinal muscular atrophy,
    145–146, 163, 164, 167,
    181
  syphilitic myelitis, 143
  syringomyelia, 141, 144–145
  tabes dorsalis, 143
  thoracic cord, 151
  transverse myclitis, 20, 143–144
  vascular disease, 147–149
Spinal hemisection, 139, 142
Spinal muscular atrophy (SMA),
    145–146, 163, 164, 167,
    181
Spinal stenosis, 139, 152
Spinal tracts, 133–135
Spinocerebellar tract, 122, 134,
    137–138
Spinomesencephalic tract, 137
Spinoreticular tract, 137
Spinothalamic tract, 66, 110–111,
    118–120, 134, 137
Spondylolisthesis, 151–152
Spondylosis, 150, 151

Sternocleidomastoid muscles,
    innervation, 105–106
Striatonigral degeneration, 55, 56
Striatum, 51–53
Stroke, 22, 47, 123
Subarachnoid hemorrhage, 13–14,
    15
Subarachnoid space, 97, 148, 152
Subcortical dementias, 43, 45–46
Subdural hematoma, 23, 148
Subdural hemorrhage, 27
Substantia nigra, 46, 51–53, 64, 66
Subthalamic nucleus, 51–53
Suck reflex, 29
Superior colliculus, 77
Superior orbital fissure syndrome,
    130
Superior temporal gyrus, 1, 66
Supramarginal gyrus, 30
Supranuclear lesions, 107
Sural nerve biopsy, 161
Swinging-flashlight test, 81, 91
Sydenham's chorea, 60, 62, 63
Syndrome of Benedikt, 108, 115
Syphilitic myelitis, 143
Syringomyelia, 141, 144–145
Syrinx, 139, 144
Systemic lupus erythematosus
    (SLE), 21, 22, 60

Tabes dorsalis, 143
Tactile sensation, 134, 138, 137
Tardive dyskinesia, 64, 65
Tarsal tunnel syndrome, 180
Taste, 66, 96
Tectospinal pathway, 138
Temporal lobe lesions, 4, 32, 37
Temporal lobe personality, 5–6, 32
Thalamic infarction, 42
Thalamic lesions, 67–69, 83

Thalamic pain syndrome, 67, 68
Thalamoperforate artery, 36, 67–68
Thalamus, 34, 65–67
Thiamine deficiency,
      encephalopathy, 11
Thoracic cord lesions, 151
Thrombosis
   basilar, 114, 130–131
   cerebral, 26
Thyroid ophthalmopathy, 91
Thyrotoxicosis, 187
Tibial neuropathy, 179–180
Tinnitus, 129
Titubation, 58
Tolosa–Hunt syndrome, 129
Tongue, 106, 107
   protrusion, 61, 62, 65
Tonic pupil, 92, 93
Top-of-the-basilar syndrome, 68,
      108, 114, 132
Torticollis, 61
Touch, 134, 138, 137, 147
Toxic encephalopathy, 10–12
Transcallosal herniation, 16
Transcortical aphasias, 39–42,
      68–69
Transverse myelitis, 20, 143–144
Trapezius muscles, innervation,
      105–106
Trauma
   brachial plexus, 173
   cauda equina, 153
   central cord syndrome, 150
   cerebral, 23, 30
   cerebral palsy, 13
   cranial nerves, 90
   diffuse cerebral edema, 13
   ocular motor muscles, 91
   tibial neuropathy, 179–180
Tremor, 55, 57–58, 59

Trigeminal nerve (CN V), 72, 80,
      94–95, 109, 115, 129, 130
Trigeminal nerve lesions, 94–95,
      129, 130
Trigeminal neuralgia, 95
Trigeminal neuropathy, 22
Trochlear nerve (CN IV), 72,
      79–80, 83, 109, 129, 130
   palsy, 14, 83, 90, 114
Trochlear nucleus, 112
Tumors
   cerebellopontine angle, 130
   cerebellum, 124–125
   cerebral, 20, 22–23
   craniocervical junction, 149
   Foster Kennedy syndrome, 128
   frontal lobe, 29
   glomus jugulare, 103
   gray matter, 140
   midbrain, 93
   olfactory groove, 29, 74
   optic nerve, 75
   Parinaud's syndrome, 114, 115
   posterior fossa, 16
   spinal cord, 141, 142
   trigeminal nerve, 94–95
Tympanic membrane, 99

Ulnar neuropathy, 173, 176

Vagus nerve (CN X), 72, 103–105,
      110, 120
   palsy, 149
Vascular claudication, legs, 152
Vascular dementia, 45
Vascular disease, 147–149
Vasculitis, 22, 161, 162, 185
Venous thrombosis, cerebral, 26
Ventral anterior (VA) nucleus,
      51–52, 66

Ventrolateral (VL) nucleus, 51–52, 66
Vergence eye movements, 75, 76
Vermis, 121–122, 125
  agenesis, 128
Vertical nystagmus, 84
Vertigo, 100–102
Vestibular apparatus, 99
Vestibular dysfunction, 100
Vestibulocochlear nerve (CN VIII), 72, 80, 99–102, 109, 110
Vestibulospinal pathways, 138
Vestibulospinal tract, 134
Ventroposterior (VP) complex, 65, 66
Ventroposterlateral (VPL) nuclei, 65
Ventropostermedial (VPM) nuclei, 66
Viral myositis, 185
Vision, 3–4; *see also* Eye movements; Ocular motor dysfunction; Ocular motor nerve; Visual field abnormalities; Visual loss
Visual field abnormalities, 32, 33
  anatomy, 46–47, 74
  cortical blindness, 33

Visual loss, 74
Visuospatial dysfunction, 49–50

Wada test, 32
Wallenberg's syndrome, 109, 120
Watershed infarcts, 13, 42
Weakness, 33–34
  cerebral cortex, 33
  differential diagnosis, 159
  facial, 97
  hypothyroidism, 188
  legs, 34, 140, 159
  muscular dystrophies, 183
  myopathies, 186–187
  syringomyelia, 144–145
Weber's syndrome, 108, 114, 115
Werdnig–Hoffman disease, 146
Wernicke's aphasia, 25, 40
Wernicke's area, 1, 25, 32, 37
Wernicke's encephalopathy, 11
White matter *see* Cerebral cortex and white matter
Wilson's disease, 60, 63
Writer's cramp, 62
Writing, 2–3